TODAY'S HERBAL HEALTH FOR CHILDREN

© 1996 Copyright

Woodland Publishing Inc.
P.O. Box 160
Pleasant Grove, UT 84062

The information contained in this book is for educational purposes only. Please consult a professional health care physician.

D1019246

DISCLAIMER

The information in this book is for educational purposes only and is not recommended as a means of diagnosing or treating an illness. All matters concerning physical and mental health should be supervised by a medical professional knowledgeable in treating that particular condition. The publisher and author neither directly nor indirectly dispense medical advice nor prescribe any remedies, natural or otherwise. They do not assume responsibility for those who choose to treat themselves.

TABLE OF CONTENTS

PART I
CHILDREN AND HEALTH

INTRODUCTION

Children are full of energy and life. They love to explore and discover things for themselves. Parents help to cultivate this awareness and excitement but also offer wisdom and control in teaching children to avoid dangerous situations. A parent has the unique responsibility of being sensitive to their child and knowing their individual needs. A parent may feel and sense when a child is not feeling quite right.

Parents want what is best for their children, and they desire to give their children an excellent start in life. Parents and children have a special bond based on love and understanding. Parents are usually the first to realize that something is wrong with their child. They recognize unusual behavior that may be the first symptom of an illness or health problem.

When a child is ill, parents want to make them well as quickly and painlessly as possible. Most often the conventional approach is taken by reaching in the medicine cabinet for quick relief or rushing to the pediatrician for a round of antibiotics. Frequently the natural methods of health and healing are overlooked. But many effective treatments are available that can help heal the body safely and naturally. In fact, these natural approaches can help the body heal itself.

This book contains information to help concerned parents learn about ways to aid the healing process, when their children are ill, using natural methods. Each treatment offers benefits. The natural approach is explained with details to

1

help the parent feel confident in taking care of their children. This book is not intended to replace conventional medical practices. But many times natural means can be used at home to heal.

PREPARING BEFORE BIRTH

Nutrition for children begins before they are born. The absence of good nutrition and adequate vitamins and minerals can affect the health of the unborn child, as well as their development. Neural tube defects in children have been linked to a deficiency of folic acid in the diet of the mother. Many doctors believe that a healthy diet may help prevent heart disease, stroke, diabetes and cancer.

PREGNANCY

When a woman becomes pregnant, or even before, nutrition is extremely important. The first month of pregnancy is crucial to the development of the fetus. The unborn child is totally dependent on its mother. The developing fetus gets all its nourishment from the mother through the placenta. The choices the mother makes in what she consumes reflects directly on the fetus. If a mother drinks alcohol, uses drugs, or smokes, the growing fetus could be affected detrimentally. It is important to make good choices right from the beginning in order to allow the best environment for growth and development of the fetus and to help ensure a strong immune system for the child.

The first few months of pregnancy are essential because of the risk of birth defects. The embryo is developing rapidly and unknown substances can affect the development. In some cases damage can occur even before the woman knows that she is pregnant. It is important to be aware and prepare the body even before thinking about becoming pregnant. Folic acid has been found to be essential in preventing neural tube defects, and zinc has been researched and found to help ensure a healthy and good-sized baby.

3

To prevent complications during pregnancy a healthy diet high in vitamins and minerals before becoming pregnant is essential. More nutrients are needed during pregnancy and most health care professionals recommend a supplement. Eat a diet high in vegetables, fruits, complex carbohydrates, and protein. A good diet can help prevent constipation, toxemia, anemia, morning sickness, fatigue and other complications. Avoid refined foods, chocolate, caffeine, sugar products, fast food, fatty foods and rancid oils. A juice fast using green drinks and other fresh juices can help clean the liver of toxins.

Herbs and herbal combinations can be safe and useful during pregnancy. Many are helpful alternatives to drugs to help with problems during pregnancy. Herbs to use during pregnancy include:

Red Raspberry: This can help relieve nausea, strengthen the uterus, clean and tone the mucus membranes, ease premature labor, and assist during labor and delivery.

Bilberry: Bilberry helps to strengthen the veins and capillaries. It also helps with kidney function and is a mild diuretic.

Burdock: Burdock helps to prevent bloating and jaundice in the baby.

Chamomile: This is a digestive aid, helps with bowel problems and induces relaxation.

Ginger: Ginger helps with digestion and nausea due to morning sickness.

Horsetail/Oatstraw: These help to provide valuable minerals to strengthen the body and fetus.

Chlorophyll: Chlorophyll is rich in nutrients to build and promote health.

Dandelion: This is high in iron and nutrients to help prevent anemia.

Kelp: Kelp is full of nutrients and easily assimilated in the

4

body. It can help strengthen the uterus and prevent anemia.

Alfalfa: Alfalfa is high in nutrients and contains vitamin K to prevent hemorrhage. It also helps with digestion and assimilation of nutrients and to purify the blood.

Slippery Elm: Slippery Elm is rich in protein and soothing on the mucous membranes.

Peppermint: Peppermint can be used after the first trimester to help with digestion and soothe the stomach.

Wild Yam: This helps prevent miscarriage, pregnancy pain, nausea and cramping.

Yellow Dock: This is high in iron and aids in building the blood. It can help to prevent infant jaundice.

Herbs to avoid during pregnancy, especially during the first trimester, include: Pennyroyal, Blue Cohosh, Black Cohosh, Squaw Vine, Spikenard, Mistletoe, False Unicorn, Angelica, Cinchona, Eucalyptus Oil, Juniper, Lovage, Ma Huang, Male Fern, Rue, Tansy, Wormwood, and Yarrow. Golden Seal should only be used in small amounts. Laxative herbs may cause stomach cramps which may lead to contractions and should be used sparingly or in combinations only. Some include Aloe Vera, Barberry, Buckthorn, Cascara Sagrada, Mandrake, Rhubarb, and Senna.

Combinations are available to be taken six weeks before delivery to help prepare the body for a healthy delivery. It may contain some or all of the following: Squaw Vine, Blessed Thistle, Black Cohosh, Pennyroyal, False Unicorn and Red Raspberry.

COMMON PREGNANCY COMPLAINTS AND HERBAL REMEDIES

Anemia: Alfalfa, Chlorophyll, Dandelion, Kelp and Yellow Dock. Vitamin C helps with the absorption of iron.

Backache: Constipation may be a problem. Bowel Formula, Chlorophyll, and a Fiber Supplement.

Constipation: Lower Bowel Formula, Fiber Supplement, and Roughage.

False Labor: Catnip and Chamomile will relax the uterus.

Gas: Starch, sugars and meat may cause fermentation. Ginger, Papaya, and Herbal Digestion Formulas.

Headache: Constipation, high blood pressure and toxemia may cause headaches. Lower Bowel Formula, Chlorophyll, Nervine Herbs such as Valerian, Hops and Chamomile.

Heartburn: Papaya, Ginger, Digestion Formulas, and B-Complex.

Hemorrhoids: Constipation contributes to the problem. Pure Water, Fiber Supplement, Bowel Formula, White Oak Bark, Fresh Lemon Juice in Pure Water, and Kelp.

High Blood Pressure: Toxins in the blood can contribute. Eliminate meat and dairy products. Eat vegetables and fruit and drink plenty of pure water. Red Clover, Blood Purifying Combinations, Chlorophyll and Green Drinks.

Hormone Imbalance: This may occur because of the excess estrogen in the blood during pregnancy. Chlorophyll, Bowel Combination and Liver Combination.

Insomnia: Calcium Herbal Formulas, Kelp, Passion Flower, Chlorophyll, Herbal Nervine Combination, Calcium and Magnesium.

Leg Cramps: Calcium, Magnesium, Calcium Herbal Formulas, Vitamins C and D.

Miscarriage: Red Raspberry Tea, Catnip Tea, Lobelia, and Sarsaparilla.

Morning Sickness: Red Raspberry Tea, Catnip, Peppermint, Spearmint, Ginger, Chlorophyll and Green Drinks.

Nervous Disorders: Calcium, Magnesium, Kelp, Vitamin C, Passion Flower, Hops, Scullcap, and Chlorophyll.

RH Negative Factor: Lower Bowel Formula, Liver Cleanser, and Blood Purifying Combination.

Stretch Marks: Vitamin A, E, Zinc, Olive Oil, and Wheat Germ Oil.

Toxemia: Vitamins C, A, B-Complex and E, Fresh Lemon Juice in Water, Green Drinks and Chlorophyll. Eliminate red meat, salt and sugar. Add fresh vegetables, fruits and whole grains.

Urinary Tract Infections: Vitamin C, Pure Water, Parsley Tea, Green Drinks, Chlorophyll, Unsweetened Cranberry Juice and Herbal Urinary Combination.

Vaginal Yeast Infection: Acidophilus, Raspberry Tea, Pure Water, Vitamins A and C, and Chlorophyll.

Water Retention: Vitamin C, Parsley, and Herbal Urinary Formula.

BREAST FEEDING

Breast feeding is both natural and practical for many women. It is the preferred choice whenever possible by both the medical and natural health communities and beneficial for both mother and child. It is also a unique bonding time for mother and child as well as being the best nutritional start for a baby. It is a wonderful way to establish an environment for the total development of the child. Breast milk is adapted to meet the needs of the infant and contains all the nutrients necessary for a great start. It doesn't mean that women who are unable to breast feed are bad mothers. The most important factor is to offer a loving, peaceful environment for the newborn. There are supplements available and formulas with health in mind for bottle fed babies. But the best choice is breast feeding.

When a baby is born, the immune system is not fully formed. It is functioning, but not at full speed. Leo Galland, M.D. in his book *Super Immunity For Kids* on page 52 states, "A newborn infant's lymphocytes are also not yet capable of making all the different kinds of antibodies she needs. They acquire that ability slowly over her first year of life. The last one they begin to make is the IgA antibody, which performs a crucial service: coating her intestinal and respiratory tracts, thus protecting them against infection. Because their bodies can't yet make the IgA antibody, infants under a year are particularly prone to intestinal-tract infections." Breast milk contains substances which offer protection to the infant's intestinal tract.

Breast milk contains elements vital in protecting the infant against infections and allergies. The baby has the mother's antibodies for the first three months of life. Research has shown that formula fed babies are often less healthy than breast fed babies. They are more prone to ear infections and allergies as well as other illnesses. Breast milk contains substances to enhance the defense system of the infant. Interferon is found in breast milk and is beneficial for fighting immune-related diseases such as viral infections and maybe even cancer. Human milk contains enzymes that are advantageous in breaking down milk fat to form free fatty acids that are known to help inhibit the growth of parasites in the intestines. Breast milk is also helpful in enhancing the development of favorable bacteria such as Lactobacillus bifidus which aids in the metabolism of vitamins, minerals and amino acids and helps break down milk sugar into lactic acid.

Breast milk contains important substances that help prevent allergies in the baby. Breast feeding can help the baby develop a strong immune system. And the breast milk contains everything that the baby needs for development during the first six months of life.

PREVENTION

Prevention is the key to health. Preventive medicine is practiced in many different societies. The Asian cultures emphasize staying well and healthy more than treating the symptoms of an illness. It involves keeping the body in optimum health through nutrition, exercise, rest, and natural supplements. But even under the best of circumstances, there will be problems. Illness will occur in our less than perfect environment. Accidents will happen no matter how hard we try to avoid them. Being prepared and knowledgeable can make things easier when problems do occur.

Children will become ill. It is important for them to experience common ailments in order to help develop and strengthen their immune systems. A cold or flu is nature's way of eliminating toxins from the body. No child is immune from the toxins that are in the environment. Most childhood diseases respond to the body's normal defense system.

Prevention actually begins while the fetus is developing inside the mother. The health of the baby rests to a great extent on what the mother ingests. The mother is responsible for nourishing the growing baby through the placenta. If the baby is given a good start nutritionally from conception, he will have a greater chance of being born with a strong immune system. A pregnant woman should take a nutrient supplement because of the needs and demands of the fetus. Pregnant women need to take a supplement containing vitamin C, B-complex, calcium, magnesium, and zinc. The pregnant woman should eat well, not trying to diet during her pregnancy, to produce a healthy child with a strong immune system. Meals should be eaten regularly.

NUTRITION BASICS

It is impossible to prescribe a correct diet which will work for every child. And there are certainly contradictory theories concerning all types of nutritional regimens. Diets and nutritional information abound. Some claim a high protein diet is the answer. Others swear by a high fiber, low carbohydrate routine. And some recommend high amounts of complex carbohydrates. But it is important to use common sense. Consider your child's individual needs. Different amounts of nutrients are needed for children at different times in their lives. Proper nutrition is an important contributing factor in the total health of a child's body. And it is necessary to pay attention to what is actually being consumed. Nutrients are divided into three basic categories. They include fats, carbohydrates, and protein.

FATS

Fats are the most calorie-dense nutrient. They are made of carbon, hydrogen, and oxygen. Fats contain nine calories per gram. This is almost twice that found in carbohydrates and protein.

The human body needs fat in the diet to survive. But the amount needed is very small in relation to the overall diet. Many children enjoy foods high in fat. With the pace of life most of us live, we often choose to feed our children fast food which is usually high in fat. This life style full of high-fat foods is not good for a child's body. High-fat diets are responsible for contributing to many illnesses and disorders, including some types of cancer, cardiovascular disease, intestinal problems, hypertension, and autoimmune diseases.

A small amount of fat is essential to a healthy body. A

layer of fat insulates the body from the environment. Fat-soluble vitamins, A, D, E, and K, need dietary fat to be utilized by the body. Linoleic acid found in polyunsaturated fats such as grains, nuts, seeds, and some vegetables help the body metabolize fats. Fats are needed by the body cells to help perform many vital roles including brain function, the production of certain hormones, nerve impulses, and metabolism. And some forms of dietary fat such as linoleic acid, eicosapentaenoic acid, and linolenic acid all contribute to vital functions. Fats are important to a child's body; however, excess fat in the diet is detrimental to a child's health.

Most of dietary fat falls under one of three categories of fatty acids which are saturated, polyunsaturated, and monounsaturated. Most animal fat is composed of saturated fats. And most vegetable, seed, and nut oils consist of polyunsaturated and monounsaturated fatty acids.

Saturated fats are considered to be the least healthy for the body. Their composition causes them be become hard when refrigerated. The major contributor to saturated fats is animal fat. But some vegetable oils such as coconut and palm oils are also high in saturated fat. Evidence is clear that a diet high in saturated fats can lead to many health problems. In cultures where there is little availability of saturated fats in the diet, there are few cases of coronary heart disease. In our American culture, the consumption of saturated fats is high. And we certainly see the results in the high number of individuals suffering from heart disease and atherosclerosis. A diet low in saturated fats is encouraged.

Polyunsaturated fats are usually recommended over saturated. But they also can cause problems. A theory known as the free radical theory states that certain areas of unsaturation in the chain of fatty acids are very vulnerable to attack by oxygen when exposed to the air, especially when heated. This can release free radicals and peroxides. The free radicals are responsible for changing more of the fats to peroxides, and the peroxides cause the production of more free radicals. These free radicals are very destructive and can cause damage to DNA and lead to cancer and premature aging. Polyunsaturated fats when used rather than saturated fats, are known to help lower cholesterol levels. Butter is thought to cause less damage because of its lower amounts of free radicals released when heated. So what is the answer? Probably a lower intake of all types of fats and choosing to use monounsaturated oils in small amounts.

Monounsaturated fats are considered by many to be the best to use in moderation. These include olive oil and canola oil. Considerable studies have been done using olive oil. It seems that olive oil is beneficial in lowering LDL cholesterol levels and not in lowering the HDL cholesterol levels, which are beneficial and protective. Olive oils which are not refined are usually recommended because of their protection against oxidation and the release of free radicals.

A diet low in overall fat consumption is highly recommended, and using monounsaturated oils whenever possible in moderation. Small amounts of other fats may be consumed on a limited basis. The diet should not consist of more than 20 to 30 % of the calories in the form of fat. The ideal to shoot for is probably in the 10 to 15 % range. But it is important that children do need fat in their diets for proper growth and development. Remember to read the labels of products to learn the fat content.

The hydrogenation process involves vegetable and seed oils going through an elaborate process to saturate the carbon molecules with hydrogen. This is done by heating to temperatures up to 410 degrees under high pressure with a metal catalyst such as nickel, platinum and copper. A liquid oil can be changed by this process to a solid or semi-solid state such as in margarine or shortenings. The nutritional value is lost in the process, and it may contain harmful chemicals altered during the process. There may be traces of

13

harmful metals. Trans fatty acids, left behind in the process, are known to be harmful and interfere with body functions.

CHOLESTEROL

Cholesterol is a term that we are all familiar with. It brings fear into the minds of many. But it is a necessary component for synthesizing vitamin D, hormones produced in the adrenal glands and for the reproductive organs. The liver will make the cholesterol necessary if it is not eaten in the diet. There are actually two types of cholesterol; low-density lipoproteins, or LDL which is considered the bad cholesterol, and high-density lipoproteins, or HDL which is thought to be the good cholesterol.

LDL cholesterol is the type that can cause damage to the artery walls. It contains a chemical known as apolipoprotein B which is responsible for the problems. It is a wax like substance which can accumulate in the arteries adhering to the arterial walls often near the heart. The LDL cholesterol, along with the apolipoprotein B, can adhere to the arterial walls causing plaque build up and allowing less blood to flow smoothly. When the adherence is near the heart, the individual is at risk of developing coronary heart disease.

HDL cholesterol is thought to be the good cholesterol. It is considered to be beneficial in protecting the arteries. It may actually protect the cholesterol from adhering to the arterial walls. A high HDL level is helpful in preventing heart disease.

Cholesterol is a substance which circulates through the body. It is controlled by the liver which can aid in removing the cholesterol from the blood and returning it to bile which aids in digestion. In the bile, the cholesterol can again be absorbed back into the bloodstream. The total cholesterol count is important because of the ratio between the HDL and the LDL.

Cholesterol count is affected by different factors. Heredity is thought to play a major role in cholesterol levels. Children who eat diets high in fat and cholesterol are at higher risk of developing high cholesterol levels. There are a few who can get away with it due to highly efficient liver function. Many children have been found to be in the early stages of heart disease because of a poor diet. Following the basic nutritional guidelines by eating a diet rich in vegetables, fruit, and whole grains will aid in controlling cholesterol levels. Exercise and stress management are also effective tools in lowering overall cholesterol levels in the blood.

CARBOHYDRATES

In the past, Carbohydrates were thought to be largely responsible for problems with obesity. Experts recommended limiting all carbohydrates and starchy food to lose weight. But times have changed and this basic food group is known to be essential to health and weight loss.

The sugar in the carbohydrates are used for energy. All carbohydrates consist of one or more simple sugars. One is called a monosaccharide. When two combine, it is known as a disaccharide. And a combination of more than two simple sugars is called a polysaccharide. The polysaccharides are also known as complex carbohydrates.

Simple carbohydrates are found in the form of different sugars including glucose, fructose, sucrose, and lactose. Complex carbohydrates, commonly known as starches, are essential to health. They consist of whole grain products, rice, potatoes, pasta, corn, etc. These complex carbohydrates are important to the body and are a valuable source of energy.

They are easily utilized as energy for the body. They are usually low in calories. It's the added fat and sugar that cause problems.

When the carbohydrates are refined (such as white flour and rice), they lose their value. They can still serve as a source of energy, but fiber and vital nutrients are lost in the processing. It is important to include whole grain products to ensure a healthy diet.

Simple sugars are burned immediately by the body. This can cause large fluctuations in blood sugar levels when large amounts are consumed. Insulin is required to remove the glucose from the blood. And this results in a sharp lowering of the blood sugar levels. The starches or complex carbohydrates take longer to digest and do not cause the same fluctuations. The body can store the starches and use the calories as needed.

Some forms of sugar considered natural include fructose, maple sugar, date sugar, honey and raw brown sugar. They still cause some blood sugar level fluctuations. Some may contain small amounts of vitamins and minerals, but they should still be used in moderation.

PROTEIN

Protein is found abundantly in the body. It contributes to many important functions in the body. Protein helps with the growth and repair of tissue in the body including muscle and bone. They also help make up the complex cell structure.

Protein is broken down through the digestion process into amino acids. There are many different combinations of amino acids in the body. Twenty-two of these are considered important for life. Eight of these cannot be manufactured from other amino acids and are considered essential amino acids.

They must come from the diet on a daily basis.

Only a small amount of protein is needed in the diet. And most individuals get much more than the four ounces a day needed to sustain life. The excess is burned as energy. But protein is not considered to be an efficient source of energy. Protein involves a complex combination of molecules. It takes longer for the body to digest and use this energy. High amounts of protein in the body put extra stress and work on the digestive system, contributing to feelings of fatigue. Protein contains nitrogen which must be eliminated from the body through the work of the liver and kidneys. This is stressful on those organs of the body.

Proteins in the form of legumes, vegetables, and grains do not contain all the essential amino acids. But by combining incomplete proteins, all the essential amino acids can be consumed.

Protein should be eaten in moderation from meat sources, especially those high in saturated fat such as red meat. Poultry contains less fat especially when the and skin is removed. Fish is a good source of protein but be careful of contamination. Eggs are high in protein.

Legumes, which include peas, beans, lentils, and soy products, are good sources of protein. Whole grain products contain some protein. They can be eaten with other protein foods. Nuts and seeds are high in protein but also contain high amounts of fat.

Complete proteins in a given day can be supplied by these combinations: corn and beans; rice and beans; grains and legumes; grains and seeds; or seeds and legumes. Of course, varying amounts of amino acids are found in most natural foods. Avoiding junk food and concentrating on nutritious foods can ensure the body's efficient utilization of protein.

If complementary proteins are eaten throughout the day, the body can assimilate them and extract the amino acids it needs to fulfill the daily requirements needed. Protein from plant sources can be more easily assimilated than the protein found in meats. Protein requirements can be met if a wide variety of vegetables, grain, legumes, fruits, and a little meat are consumed.

The synthetic hormones found in animal products such as milk, cheese, eggs, and meat can cause problems. Excessive estrogen from these sources, when not eliminated by the liver, can lead to breast cancer, as well as cancer of the reproductive system and many other problems. Precocious puberty is one condition found in children which is linked to excess hormone consumption. Too much protein from animal sources may cause problems such as constipation, autotoxemia, hyperactivity, nutritional deficiencies, kidney damage, heart disease, and cancer.

The most important information to remember is to eat a nutritionally balanced diet including ample amounts of complex carbohydrates, some protein, and just a little fat.

ENZYMES

Enzymes are the protein-like substances formed in plants and animals. They act as catalysts in chemical reactions. Enzymes speed up the processes in the body.

Glands and organs in the body depend on the activity of the enzymes to function properly Enzymes are found in all living things. There are around 700 different enzymes which function in the body. They each perform a different role. Enzymes supply energy for the body and are found in raw, live food. This includes fresh fruits and vegetables. When the valuable enzymes are missing in the body, the glands must try and manufacture the ones it needs. This can cause the glands to overwork and cause feelings of fatigue and exhaustion.

There are four main categories of food enzymes. These include:

1. Lipase (which serves to break down fat)

2. Protease (which breaks down protein)

3. Cellulase (which assists in breaking down cellulose)

4. Amylase (which breaks down starch)

AMINO ACIDS

Amino acids are considered the building blocks of protein. Proteins are substances which occur in all living matter. A proper balance of amino acids can benefit the blood, skin, immune system, and digestive system. Amino acids also can help with neurotransmitters in the brain, helping to stabilize moods and balance nerve transmissions in the brain.

There are eight essential amino acids and twenty-four complementary ones which work synergistically to promote health in the body. Carnitine is an example of an amino acid which helps to metabolize fat and reduce triglycerides. Carnitine is synthesized from the combination of the amino acids lysine and methionine. Methionine helps remove heavy metals from the tissue. Lead, mercury, aluminum, arsenic, cadmium are some heavy metals which can cause brain damage as well as serious illness.

FIBER

Fiber has come to the public's attention through medical advice and the media. It is certainly an important item that was neglected for a period of time and considered non-essential. In fact, it was removed from foods to make them smooth and more appetizing. Fiber was thought to have no nutritional benefits. But times have changed and more and more people are realizing the healthy contribution fiber can make in their diets. Fiber has always been considered important in the natural nutritional world. When processed foods were introduced, individuals became attracted to their convenience and taste. But now more attention is being placed on fiber and its importance. And this is one area in which the medical community and natural health field agree.

Fiber constitutes of the cell walls of plants. Plants are supported by these that keep them rigid. Every plant cell has a wall of fibers. It is usually considered to be the parts of the foods we eat that are not digestible. However, this is the material that is important in keeping the digestive process moving and the intestinal system functioning efficiently.

Insoluble fibers absorb water, swelling and adding bulk. Some of these include celluloses, lignins, and hemicelluloses found in whole grains and vegetables. Water-soluble fibers are found in apples, citrus fruits, oats, legumes, and some vegetables. They are known as gums, pectins, and mucilages.

Studies have been conducted, making fantastic claims to the importance of fiber. Lower cholesterol levels have been attributed to fiber intake as well as the prevention of heart disease and colon cancer. The important thing to remember is that most people do not get enough fiber. The National Cancer Institute has recommended that people eat at least 20 to 35 grams of fiber each day. And many experts suggest as much as 40 grams per day. The average American probably only consumes around 10 to 15 grams of fat per day.

In cultures where fruits, vegetables, and whole grains are eaten in abundance, there is less incidence of obesity, colitis, cancer, polyps of the colon, and appendicitis. Experts attribute this to the high fiber content contained in the diets of these people. The fiber adds bulk and also the elimination time is increased, speeding up the process. It seems that the quicker the food is eliminated through the system, the greater the benefits. Fiber can keep the toxins from building up in the colon by keeping the bowels moving. Proteins and fats are absorbed mainly in the intestines. This may lead to constipation problems. The theory is that the less time toxins and carcinogenic substances remain in the bowels, the less chance of them causing problems. Diets low in dietary fiber allow the food to remain longer in the intestines causing toxins to build up which may lead to the beginning of disease. The fiber will not cure cancer, but it may help in preventing problems for susceptible individuals. Also cholesterol and fats are excreted from the body at a faster pace as well as toxins. A high fiber diet can help the bowel wall remain strong, clean and healthy.

Fiber is often lacking in children's diets. The best method of increasing fiber in a child's diet is to include whole grains, brown rice, oats, pasta, and ample amounts of fruits and vegetables. Be aware of what your child is eating. Fast foods are not only high in fat, but very low in fiber. Fiber should be gradually introduced into the diet to avoid intestinal problems such as diarrhea, bloating, and flatulence, (gas).

ESSENTIAL FATTY ACIDS

Essential Fatty Acids are crucial to the health of a child's immune system. They cannot be made in the body and must be acquired by the food eaten or in supplements. They are found in certain nut oils, seeds and fish. Processed oils have been depleted of the Essential Fatty Acids for the most part.

The EFA's are separated into two categories. One is the omega-6 group found mainly in seeds such as safflower, sunflower, corn oils and evening primrose oil. The group of EFA's that are usually lacking in a child's diet are the omega-3 EFA's. These can be found in flaxseed oil, soybean, walnut, wheat germ oils, cod-liver oil and cold water fish such as salmon, tuna, mackerel, herring and sardines. Dried beans such as kidney and navy contain both types of EFA's. Processing and cooking can destroy the EFA's.

The Essential Fatty Acids are important for carrying fat-soluble vitamins, A, D, E, and K. They help reduce cholesterol levels and regulate blood pressure. They are necessary for immune system function, growth and the development of healthy skin, hair and nails.

INDOLES

Indoles are some of the phytochemicals found in vegetables. They increase the activity of enzymes that can detoxify carcinogens and may also change the hormone estrogen into benign forms, reducing the risk of breast cancer and other types of cancer. Scientists think that the indoles have the ability to block cancer causing substances before they enter the cells. They are found in abundance in cruciferous vegetables. They don't seem to participate in normal functions of the body, but they do help the immune system in fighting disease. Indoles are found in some children's supplements along with vitamins and minerals to help strengthen the body, improve nutrition and prevent disease.

SUGAR AND SWEETENERS

There are many forms of sugar, both raw and refined. Food must taste good to sell, and so sugar has become a popular additive to many commercial foods. Sugar is an easy way to make food taste good and most children are hooked. All forms of sugar belong to the carbohydrate family. They all have similar molecular structures which include a carbon atom attached to hydrogen and oxygen.

The body makes glucose by breaking down carbohydrate foods. Such as fruits, vegetables, and grains. Complex carbohydrates are the greatest source of energy for the body. They are necessary for the process of digestion and the assimilation of nutrients taken into the body.

Digestion changes carbohydrates into glucose. This glucose goes to the pancreas where the increase in the blood glucose level stimulates the production of insulin. The insulin is carried by the bloodstream to the liver where the excess glucose is converted to glycogen which is stored in the liver until the liver is full to capacity.

If the insulin supplied by the pancreas is too great, too much glucose will be converted to glycogen. The blood glucose level will remain low. This is known as hypoglycemia. This is caused by eating too many simple sugars.

When the pancreas supplies too little insulin, the liver cannot convert excess glucose to glycogen. This condition is diabetes. The pancreas wears out from producing insulin to neutralize sugar foods. Sugar builds up in the blood and the blood glucose level rises and remains high.

Sugar robs the body of valuable nutrients. When sugar is eaten often and in excess, the body produces an acidic condition. In this acidic state more and more minerals are required to keep the body in balance. The body uses calcium from the bones which leaves the body (including the teeth) in a weakened condition. This is especially detrimental for children who need calcium for growth and development of the body structural system. To metabolize refined sugar, the body finds the missing nutrients from other sources. These can be from foods eaten in the same meal or from the body tissue itself. We lose vitamins and minerals, especially vitamin B, calcium, phosphorous and iron from our own body reserve.

Sugar is eaten in excess by many American children. It is one of the most destructive elements in our diets. It acts as a drug and is very addictive. The more you eat the more you crave. These cravings can be satisfied with vegetables, fruits and grains. Some sweeteners seem to be absorbed slower and may cause less havoc in the body. Some sweeteners also contain nutrients and do not deplete the body of it's own resources.

Sucrose is refined white sugar or common table sugar. It is made from sugar cane and sugar beets. When sugar cane and sugar beets are refined, the result is almost pure sucrose. Each sucrose molecule is made of one fructose molecule and one dextrose molecule. Americans consume about 100-140 pounds of this white sugar per year. Sucrose contains no protein, minerals or vitamins. It is almost 100% pure simple carbohydrate. It quickly turns to glucose in the body.

Raw sugar is brown in color. This color means that some nutrients remain. It is in a granular form. Raw sugar is obtained from the evaporation of sugar cane juice. This sugar is then refined and produces white sugar or sucrose.

Brown sugar is made of sugar crystals in a molasses syrup with natural flavor and color. Most of the brown sugar in the United States simply consists of white refined sugar with a little molasses added for color. A small amount of nutrients are added to the refined sugar through the molasses.

Corn syrup is produced by adding enzymes to cornstarch. High fructose corn syrup comes from corn. The amount of fructose in the corn syrup will vary between manufacturers. And the rest of the corn syrup is dextrose. It is used as a sweetener often to prevent other sugars from forming crystals when they cool.

Dextrose is the same as glucose. It is made from synthetic starch by the action of heat and enzymes.

Lactose is milk sugar. It occurs naturally in the milk of all mammals. It is made from whey.

Fructose is also known as levulose. It is a commercially produced sugar which has the same molecular structure as fructose naturally found in fruit and honey. It is made from sucrose which is composed of fructose and glucose. So basically, the glucose is taken out which leaves the fructose. Studies have supported the belief that fructose does not seem to stimulate insulin production by the pancreas. When fructose enters the bloodstream, it does not seem to require insulin to get into the cells. Some of the fructose is metabolized in the liver. Some portions of fructose are converted to glycogen which eventually is changed to glucose and does require insulin. But this is a much slower process and causes the glucose to enter the bloodstream at a slow and even rate. Fructose is thought by many to not cause the large fluctuations in blood glucose levels and causes less stress on the pancreas than sucrose.

Blackstrap molasses is the syrup that remains after sugar is crystallized out of sugar cane juice. The process is repeated many times to get all the color and nutrients out. Molasses is the residue that contains the minerals and vitamins from sugar cane. Blackstrap molasses contains calcium, phosphorus, iron, sodium, potassium, thiamine, riboflavin, and niacin. It can be used, in some cases, as a sugar substitute.

Honey is a complex sugar consisting mainly of fructose and glucose with some minerals and vitamins. It contains no protein or fat. Honey varies in flavor, depending on what flower nectar it is from. It contains different sugars from the nectar as well as additives from the bee's digestive system. These work as a preservative which allows honey to keep for a long period of time. Honey is absorbed slower than other sugars because of its high fructose content.

Studies have shown that bacteria cannot grow in honey because of its potassium content. This mineral absorbs the liquid in which the bacteria need to survive. It can be used to prevent infections. It is soothing to the skin tissue and has been used effectively as a treatment for burns. Honey has been used as a folk remedy. It is a great tasting alternative to other sweeteners.

Maple syrup is found in three different grades. Grade A is mild tasting and sweet but contains less minerals. Grade B has more minerals and maple taste. Grade C is the highest in minerals but has a very strong maple taste. The vitamin and mineral content varies, depending on where the syrup is from.

Some experts feel that there is no special advantage to eating any specific type of sugar. There are some differences, but they can all cause problems when used in extreme amounts. Remember to use moderation when using sugar in all forms. It is important to pay attention to your sugar intake no matter what form it is in. This includes fruit, fruit juices, ice cream, candy or prepared foods.

ARTIFICIAL SWEETENERS

There is a lot of controversy regarding the use of artificial sweeteners. Many support the belief that these sweeteners have many advantages over natural forms of sugar. But studies seem to suggest that they should not be a part of a child's diet or used during pregnancy and breast feeding.

NutraSweet® and Equal® are the trade names for aspartame. Advocates claim that aspartame is naturally made from two building blocks of protein similar to those found in fruits, vegetables, grains, and dairy products. But others claim that this product is far from natural. It is composed of two amino acids which are phenylalanine and aspartic acid and found in nature. But the problem seems to be that they are isolated from the other amino acids with which they usually are found in combination. And the two amino acids that aspartame does contain are delivered in the body in a highly concentrated form which the body does not ordinarily have to metabolize.

Artificial sweeteners are hundreds of times sweeter than sugar. And some researchers believe that the body is tricked into thinking it is getting a large amount of sugar. This causes the metabolic process to speed up, leaving the individual hungry and tired. And this in return may cause more food to be eaten. Some studies have shown that dieters who use artificial sweeteners may actually gain more weight than those eating regular sugar products.

Robert K. Cooper Ph.D. states in his book *Health and Fitness Excellence* on page 340, "Don't rely on artificially sweetened foods and beverages to help you lose weight or prevent fat gain. According to an ongoing study by the American Cancer Society involving more than 78,000 women aged fifty to sixty-nine, long-term users of artificial sweeteners are more likely to gain weight than nonusers over the course of one year. In addition, fake sweeteners usually don't satisfy hunger. A recent study on aspartame conducted at Leeds University in England reported that not only was this sweetener generally ineffective in suppressing appetite, but in some people it actually increased feelings of hunger. In contrast, sugar (glucose) was found to reduce hunger and produce a feeling of fullness."

Information has brought to light new facts about aspartame. The amino acid phenylalanine is known to cause problems with some of the brain neurotransmitters. It seems to affect some levels of amino acids and the production and release of some neurotransmissions. This could alter many different brain functions causing brain damage as well as problems with blood pressure, appetite, and mood changes. Studies also suggest that aspartame could be toxic to newborns causing them to be hyperexcitable. Growing children do not need to eat anything that might causes problems for their brain function.

There are also some who have claimed other side affects associated with the use of aspartame. These include dizziness, nausea, diarrhea, headaches, seizures, and mood changes. Reports have been sent to the National Center for Disease Control concerning this issue. And the company responsible has also been sent many complaints.

Cyclamates, were banned some years ago, but are now being reconsidered. Saccharin is known to cause cancer and still present as an artificial sweetener.

Most natural health advocates recommend using natural sugar in small amounts and staying away from artificial sweeteners. There is really no evidence to support the use of artificial sweeteners as beneficial. And it would be wise for children as well as pregnant and nursing women to avoid products containing aspartame.

NUTRITION / BUILDING THE IMMUNE SYSTEM

THE IMMUNE SYSTEM / THE BODY'S BEST DEFENSE

The immune system is the body's best defense against disease. So it is important to strengthen the immune system in children to keep them as healthy as possible. The immune system consists of various cells with specific responsibilities throughout the body which have the ability to recognize and destroy substances that can be harmful. They try to neutralize and destroy foreign substances that can invade the body. Some members of the immune system include white blood cells, the lymph system, immunoglob-ulins, interferon and interleukin. Each immune cell serves a specific function. Some know how to locate and attack antigens in the body and others must receive instructions to work. The white blood cells or leukocytes play a major role in fighting the battle against invaders. They are aided by other members of the immune system.

The key to prevention is to start when children are young to improve immune function. The immune system can become damaged gradually over many years of abuse. The problems can build up, starting out as minor discomfort and becoming more severe. All children are exposed to toxins each day while at home, school or outdoor playing. These toxins will affect children differently, depending on the condition of their immune systems. The immune system helps eliminate toxins and fight infections and disease. A wholesome, natural diet, natural supplements and exercise can help keep the immune system working well.

Surface immunity problems occur in everyone. These

include the common cold, flu, acute infections and allergies. These usually are minor and short lived and are the body's method of getting rid of built-up toxins. If the immune system is in good condition, the body will heal quickly. More severe disorders can occur when the body's immune system is weak, under stress or has suffered long-term abuse. The immune cells are created in the bone marrow and these reserves can become depleted, leaving the body more susceptible to various disorders. Some of these more severe reactions to a weak immune system include: AIDS, cancer, leukemia, tumors, allergies, Reye's syndrome, Lupus, mental problems, and chemical imbalances.

Aspirin irritates the stomach and intestines. This can hinder the ability of the intestines to absorb nutrients and can lead to anemia. It can also cause birth defects when taken during pregnancy, cause internal bleeding, lead to allergies and kidney damage. Aspirin can hinder the immune function and has also been linked to Reye's syndrome.

Antibiotics and vaccinations can weaken the immune system. The white blood cells become weak when antibiotics are used, leaving the body more susceptible to other problems. The body will reduce production of immune fighting cells. When children require antibiotic therapy or vaccinations are given, immune-building supplements should be given.

Sugar can also hinder immune function. It fills the stomach and replaces the necessary nutrients for health. Children who eat large quantities of sugar are less likely to eat nutritious food when it is offered. Encourage good eating habits early in life to strengthen the immune system.

NUTRITION

The most important factor in strengthening the immune system is proper nutrition. Often, parents rely on their pediatrician to tell them what their child should eat. After all, they have been trained for many years in treating children, but medical professionals usually have very little nutritional training during their educational experience. It is important to research what is best for children to eat. Look for whole and natural foods for the most nutritional value.

Eating a variety of foods will help the body get the nutrients that it needs and also make mealtime more enjoyable. Whenever possible, buy organically grown produce and grains. Buy meat from animals that have not been treated with antibiotics and hormones that can be dangerous to children. There are a wide variety of fruits and vegetables available in the supermarket which are nutritious and delicious. Fresh fruits and vegetables are full of nutrients. Canned, dried, and frozen foods often lose some of their nutritional value through the processing procedure. Additives also can be undesirable. Remember to wash thoroughly or peel produce that has been treated with pesticides.

One study found that eating too much cooked food and little raw food can overwork the immune system. The white blood cells in the intestines increase after eating cooked foods. Cooked food appears to put a strain on the immune system. When eating raw foods, the white blood cells stay the same. Giving children plenty of raw fruits and vegetables can help the immune system by providing essential nutrients and enzymes.

VEGETABLES AND FRUITS

Vegetables and fruits are important to a balanced and nutritional diet for all children. They are full of vitamins, minerals, enzymes, protein, complex carbohydrates, and fiber. There are many different varieties available.

If possible, it is important to buy produce that is free of pesticides. Or grow as much produce as possible to ensure quality and safety. Produce from local farmers can be used to be sure of the freshness.

Try and introduce new types of produce to children. If they refuse the new food, keep offering it to them. Some children need to adjust to new foods gradually before they are willing to try them. There are many exotic and different varieties available at the local supermarket. Prepare them in different ways such as shapes.

Raw as well as cooked vegetables should be included in the diet. Some should be cooked to make sure that the natural toxins are eliminated. These include broccoli, collards, kale, and Brussels sprouts. Carrots, onions, garlic, salad greens, cucumbers, radishes, peppers, and tomatoes are great eaten raw. Again, variety is the key. Vegetables are essential to a healthy body.

Fruits should be sun-ripened if possible. Unfortunately they are usually picked green and allowed to ripen on the way to the grocery store. This does not allow for the optimum amount of nutrients. Using produce from the local farmer makes it possible to acquire sun ripened fruit.

WHOLE GRAINS

More and more research and the medical community are pointing to the benefits of a diet rich in whole grain products. Processed foods are slowly losing their attractiveness in the eyes of many consumers. Whole wheat bread sales are on the rise. And there are a variety of delicious and nutritious grains available. It is now known that whole grains are important to ensure a nutritionally sound diet. They are best when grown organically to avoid contamination and pesticides. Grains can be cooked, sprouted, and ground into flour to make baked goods. Grains should not be introduced into the diet of a baby until molars have developed. This is a sign that the teeth necessary to chew and stimulate the action of enzymes required to digest the grains are available.

Grains are known to be low in fat and rich in complex carbohydrates. They have been used by many people in many cultures as a staple in the diet. They can be used to make all kinds of wonderful recipes. And they are a low cost source of nutrition, fiber, vitamins, and minerals.

Whole wheat is probably the best known grain in our culture. It is full of nutritional value. It is most often used for baking bread. Some use wheat in recipes as a meat substitute. And whole wheat can be used in soups and as a cereal. Most children are accustomed to the white flour which is the processed form of whole wheat. Unfortunately, the fiber and germ are eliminated in the processing. The whole grain wheat is a valuable nutrient.

Millet is a grain that has been used in many cultures. It is the only grain that is considered to be a complete protein. It can be added to cereals and breads and combined with other grains. It is a nutritious grain that can be introduced to babies. It can also be combined and cooked with brown rice.

Brown rice is a nutritious addition to the diet. Brown rice

needs to cook longer than white rice but the wait is worth the time. Most children are used to the white rice commonly used. But brown rice can be introduced and enjoyed by most everyone. A little butter and honey can sweeten the taste of the rice . It is full of nutritional value.

Buckwheat is a valuable grain. It is used as the main grain product in many northern European countries. The seeds of the buckwheat flower are ground into flour to make cereal and pancakes. Buckwheat is a hardy grain and it thrives in adverse conditions. It has few problems with insects and diseases and it seems to do well, even in poor soil.

Barley is a wonderful and nutritious addition to soups and stews. It is a member of the same family as corn, oats, rice, and wheat. Barley flour is used in bread, cereal and as a thickening agent.

Corn is the only vegetable that is also considered a grain. Ground corn is great for muffins, tortillas, cereal and breads. It is also used as livestock feed and to make nonfood items such as drugs, paints, and paper goods. There are several thousand different types and varieties of corn.

Oat is a very important grain. The seeds of the plant are used in oatmeal, cookies, breads, and cereals. Oats have a high food value. The majority of the crop grown in the United States is fed to livestock. But oats are becoming more popular with the interest in the health benefits of whole grain oats and oat bran.

Rye is similar to wheat. Rye is used to make delicious breads. It is thought to have been cultivated from wild species found in Asia. Rye does not contain as much gluten as wheat and is preferred by some for this reason.

LEGUMES, NUTS AND SEEDS

Legumes include peas, beans, and lentils. They are an inexpensive and nutritious addition to the diet. They contain complex carbohydrates, fiber, protein, vitamins, and minerals. They are low in fat and cholesterol.

Nuts and seeds are recommended only in small amounts because of their high fat content. They are a good source of protein and fiber and contain some essential fatty acids, vitamins, and minerals.

SUPPLEMENTS TO STRENGTHEN THE IMMUNE SYSTEM

Vitamin A/Beta-Carotene: These work as antioxidants to inhibit free radical damage and strengthen the immune system.

Vitamin C: Vitamin C is also an antioxidant and helps protect against immune-related diseases such as colds, flu and cancer.

Vitamin E: Vitamin E is an added boost for the immune system because of its ability to help produce cells to fight infection.

B-Vitamins: These help maintain a healthy nervous system to cope with tension and stress.

Selenium and Zinc: These are important for the immune system.

Rose Hips: Rose Hips contain nutrients to strengthen the immune system.

Echinacea: Echinacea is a natural antibiotic and helps to stimulate immune system function.

Capsicum: Capsicum helps to improve circulation.

Fennel: Fennel helps to stabilize the nervous system.
Garlic: Garlic is a natural antibiotic to help with infections and build the immune system to prevent disease.

FOOD ADDITIVES AND PESTICIDES

Processed foods are often full of chemicals and additives designed to prolong shelf life, improve taste and texture, and add color. Mass production has led to multiple additives being used in different foods. These food additives are tested but only on an individual basis. Animals are usually given high doses of only one single additive. In one animal study published in the *Journal of Food Sciences*, 1976, rats were given three different, common food additives. Within two weeks the rats had died. It appears that multiple additives are more detrimental.

Children are more likely to have problems from the additives because they are smaller and consume more food per body weight than adults. What may be safe for an adult, could be harmful to a small child. Most of the safety tests are done using adults without taking children into consideration.

Janet Zand, LAc, OMD, Rachel Walton, RN and Bob Roundtree MD state in their book *Smart Medicine For a Healthier Child* on pages 42-43, "A 1987 study released by the National Cancer Institute showed that children living in homes where pesticides are routinely used are seven times more likely to develop childhood leukemia than are children living in chemical-free households. In 1989, the National Resources Defense Council (NRDC) reported on a comprehensive two-year study of the impact of pesticide residues in food on children. It showed that, compared to adults, the average child receives four times more exposure to eight cancer-causing pesticides in food. Apples, apple products, peanut butter, and processed cherries that have been treated with the chemical growth regulator daminozide (better known as Alar) were named as foods posing the greatest potential risk to children. The average exposure of a child under six to daminozide and to UMDH, the carcinogenic compound it forms in the body, is 240 times the cancer risk that the Environmental Protection Agency (EPA) calls "acceptable" after a lifetime of exposure to this toxic chemical.

The study determined that children consume proportionally more fruits and vegetables, and thus more pesticides, than adults. Fruits are especially susceptible to pesticide contamination. On average, produce accounts for about one-third of a child's diet, with fruits predominating. The average preschool child consumes six times more fruit and fruit products, and drinks eighteen times more apple juice than his parents do. During infancy, the average baby consumes thirty-one times more apple juice than adults in the household."

There have been some improvements on pesticide and additive controls. But one major problem is when produce is shipped in from foreign countries which do not have the same restrictions as the United States. In fact, some American chemical companies still sell these banned additives and pesticides to foreign nations who use them on their crops.

SUGAR ADDICTION

Too much sugar in the diet of children and teenagers can create serious health problems. White sugar, (sucrose), is refined many times either from sugar cane or sugar beets. It can be acid forming and produces excess mucus in the body. Sucrose is known to leach vitamin C and B-complex vitamins from the body. Calcium and other minerals can also be robbed from the body by excess sugar consumption. The calcium, vitamins and minerals are needed for structural development and mental growth. Eating foods high in sugar can displace nutritional foods the body needs.

Sugar, in its natural state, does contain nutrients. But through the refining process, sugar is stripped of its value, and it also requires the body to provide extra amounts of enzymes and other elements for the sugar to be metabolized. Excess sugar can upset the endocrine system and cause hormone imbalances. Sugar is thought to contribute to disorders such as cancer, hormone imbalances, aggressive behavior, criminal behavior, circulatory problems, hyperactivity and degenerative diseases.

Joan Davidson, in her article "Singing Low-Down Sugar Blues", (December 1981 issue of *Chimo*) suggests, "Sugar addiction is a common factor in hypoglycemia; most people who suffer from this disease have a severe 'sweet tooth'. They crave sugar as an 'upper' because it increases their blood sugar levels and make them feel less lethargic. Like drug addiction, this is a very real problem. Anyone who has been raised on refined sugar will feel deprived if they do not have sweets or starch food for even two or three days. And like drug addiction, sugar addiction is very hard to kick. Sugar withdrawal symptoms include depression and anger and usually occur during the first two or three weeks after a change in eating habits."

Studies have been done in detention facilities to test the relationship between diet and abnormal behavior. Stephen Schoenthaler, Ph.D. and coordinator at Stanislaus State College in Turlock, California conducted research on 276 juveniles and their disruptive behavior. High sugar foods were replaced with fruit, unsweetened juices and popcorn. Antisocial behavior declined by 48%, there were 77% fewer incidents of theft, 82% less incidents of assault and 55%

reduction in refusal to obey orders. It was felt that the changes were due only to the reduction in sugar consumed. Incidentally, none of the juveniles were aware that a study was taking place. Another study conducted on fewer inmates in the Los Angeles area showed a 47% decline in fighting and aggressive behavior.

Alexander Schauss who publishes The International Journal of Biosocial Research, states in *Prevention*, October, 1983, "Excessive sugar is definitely related to deviant behavior, but it is not the only cause. The negative influence of poverty, unemployment, domestic violence and psychosocial problems cannot be discounted, but certainly vitamin deficiencies, chemical food additives, allergies, lead poisoning, iron deficiency, as well as hypoglycemia must be taken into account. I've seen prisoners use a half cup of sugar a day, juveniles about 12 ounces. This kind of overloading of sweet stuff can cause all kinds of metabolic disorders, including hypoglycemia."

A Los Angeles dentist had difficulty with an eight year old patient. He had three to five new cavities every three months. Each tooth contained a filling. He was an aggressive child who would bite, kick and scream at the dentist. Finally, the dentist recommended a sugar and white flour-free diet. The next time the boy returned, he had no cavities and his behavior had improved dramatically.

NUTRITION AND YOUTH SUICIDE

Each year over 5,000 youth attempt suicide and succeed. About 100,000 attempt suicide, and the incidences are increasing each year. A survey conducted in 1991 found that 37% of high school girls and 21% of boys had suicidal thoughts during the previous year.

Depression is the number one sign. But what causes and can be done for long term depression? Dr. Laurence Schwab, who works with youth who have attempted suicide but failed, says in *Let's Live*, January, 1984, "Doctors, psychologists, and psychiatrists who deal with suicide on a daily basis, rarely perceive that nutrition plays a powerful role in leading a person to commit suicide. Nor is credence given to the glaring signal that persons whose bodies are out of alignment—subluxated—can't think straight and might go for the shotgun, given the opportune stimulus."

Even though the youth gave many reasons for attempting suicide such as alienation from parents, no love in their lives, the end of the world, nuclear war, confusion about their place in society, living in a prison of stress, etc. Dr. Schwab discovered that one common denominator was nutrition and an imbalanced body. Sugar was often eaten in excess, the majority used caffeine and alcohol regularly, and many were involved with drugs.

The diets of the youth at risk for suicide usually consisted of junk food, caffeine drinks, white sugar products, refined foods, fast food and no supplements. Alcohol and drugs were also linked and are a cause of malnutrition and disease.

Nutrition may not be the only answer to the problem of suicide, but it can help the body handle difficult situations in a more peaceful, rational way. Children and adolescents are all subjected to stress and tension. A nutritional diet with healthy supplements can help the body deal with these stresses without resorting to extreme measures. A lack of good nutrition puts extra stress on the body.

EXERCISE

Exercise is extremely important for the development of a growing child. It is an essential part of total body health. But studies continue to show that the majority of Americans live sedentary lives. They do not participate in regular exercise. Children today are less fit and weigh more than they did 30 years ago. They spend much of their free time in front of the television. But these statistics need to change and adults, as well as children, need to become more active.

The benefits from exercise are many. A fit body is more efficient. Studies show that physical inactivity can lead to serious health problems. And some believe that a lack of exercise is responsible for many of today's health problems. Coronary heart disease, high blood pressure, high blood cholesterol levels, hypertension, strokes, and even cancer are associated in part to a lack of exercise. Exercise helps build the immune system. Children need to have fun, play time, preferably outdoors, to keep them healthy. Just as adults need exercise for health, so do children.

Regular, moderate exercise is important to good health. Experts agree that exercise can increase circulation, improve the digestive process, strengthen the heart, reduce blood pressure, increase lung capacity and oxygen utilization, lower blood cholesterol levels, and promote an overall sense of well-being, due in part to the release of endorphins. It also helps cleanse the body through perspiration, tone the nervous system, and strengthen the immune system to prevent disease.

Children need to think of exercise as fun. Adults play an important role in teaching children to enjoy physical activity by helping them to choose and participate. It is the parents' responsibility to be an example where exercise is concerned. Participating with children can be enjoyable for the whole family. Take walks, hikes, and bike rides together. Walk or ride bikes to school, activities or even shopping. Make exercise a part of life.

HERBS AND SUPPLEMENTS

Staying healthy may include supplementing the diet. When children are old enough to make some of their own food choices, and when they venture to school and activities, they may eat foods that are not allowed or encouraged at home. It is important to give them some nutritional helps through herbs and supplements.

The usual diet may contain too much fat, sugar, and protein while too little vitamins particularly B-complex, E, and C and many of the trace minerals. Adding these to a child's diet can keep them healthy and build the immune system. Look for nutritious supplements specifically for children.

HERBS FOR CHILDREN

Children can take herbs as natural supplements. Most often reduced amounts should be given to children according to their age and weight. Usually a preschool child can take about 1/4 of an adult dose. Children from ages five to ten can take about 1/2 of an adult dose. From around eleven to fifteen a dose of 3/4 the adult is recommended. When a child reaches adult size, they can take an adult dosage of herbs. Herbs can help a child develop a strong and healthy body as well as help the body heal itself of disease.

It may be difficult to get a child to take an herbal supplement. Herb powders can be added to applesauce, bananas or juices. Bitter herbs can be taken as enemas if necessary. The herbs which should be used with caution for children are the hormone herbs such as Ginseng, Damiana and Black Cohosh. These should not be used by children until they reach puberty. Laxatives such as Cascara Sagrada can be used in small dosages but may cause cramps if too much is given.

The plant kingdom has provided man with food and medicine since the beginning of time. Herbalists use the roots, flowers, leaves, stems and berries of plants to help in the treatment and prevention of illness. Herbal remedies have been used for thousands of years. Research has documented many of the traditional uses of herbal medicine. Many of the substances in the individual herbs have been isolated and found to contain healing properties. Studies are currently being done in large numbers because of the success of these herbal therapies. Herbs are used throughout the world to provide a method of treatment and the western world is slowly recognizing their benefits. For children they are a wonderful, gentle approach to healing.

Herbs are considered unique from drugs in that they contain elements in the amounts that nature intended. Drugs sometimes contain a single active substance, which has been extrapolated from a plant and synthesized. Herbs, on the other hand, provide a broad array of catalysts which work together harmoniously. They then work with the body to provide the complete healing network. Instead of focusing on an isolated segment of the human system, herbs can cleanse the entire blood supply or whatever area is affected. Herbalists believe that the natural approach using herbs can add health and vigor to the body.

Drugs made synthetically or extracted from plants are not used in a natural form. People are finding that drugs can often cause more problems than they alleviate because of side effects. Drugs are chemicals in which elements are taken from a natural source and synthesized and made stronger (an unnatural state). This new drug is in a form that is foreign to the body and may disrupt the body's internal harmony. Herbalists feel that this is the reason for side effects associated with many prescribed and over the counter drugs. Indeed, every drug contains warning labels describing possible side effects. Drugs are part of the fast paced world in which we live and demand an immediate cure to a problem. We want the doctor to prescribe a pill to rid us of the symptoms that afflict our bodies. The medical community often treats the problem, neglecting the cause of the condition. The natural approach is to look at the cause while working on healing the whole body rather than only the symptoms of an illness. In a life threatening situation, it is important to remember that any method capable of saving a life should be used. Emergencies require immediate results. There is certainly a place for the medical community in this world in which we live. And most believe that the natural methods can coexist with the modern medical therapies.

In contrast, herbs seem to be natural and safe. They do not build up in the body, producing side effects. Herbs generally contain natural buffers and synergistic substances which help balance and make the herb more useful. Herbs, as with other food, need to be used with wisdom and knowledge. Different herbs are used to help different problems. Herbs can be useful for every system of the body. Herbs are found in nature and benefit the nervous system, digestive system, circulatory system, glandular system, immune system, respiratory system, intestinal system, urinary system and the skeletal and muscular systems. The properties of each plant target specific areas of the body. Modern research has added much knowledge to the effectiveness of these herbal remedies. They are believed to contain properties which can heal and build the body. Herbs are known to be rich in vitamins and minerals which work with the body to heal specific areas.

They are a natural means of providing the body with essential nutrients which can aid in the healing process. Herbs feed the body as food does, and they work with the body to help strengthen and build up the body as it heals itself. Herbalists believe that natural herbal therapy can activate the body's own self-healing powers. This is especially good for children to help strengthen the immune system while healing.

Herbal preparations work gently and naturally to heal and strengthen the body. Children's reactions to the herbs may vary. Herbs are rarely considered toxic but should be used with caution. It is recommended to start with small amounts and observe the child's response. More may be given, if necessary. If the child shows adverse reactions to the herb, which is a rare occurrence, discontinue use.

Herbal remedies can be very beneficial for children. But getting them to take them may not be easy. They are usually unable to swallow capsules and don't like the taste of herbal teas. The tea may be added to fruit juice. Also the herbal extracts often contain glycerine which adds a slightly sweet taste to the product, making it easier to swallow. The powdered herbs can be mixed in applesauce to make them more appetizing for children. Many reputable herb companies are now adding children's supplements to their product lines. This is a great addition and worthwhile for all those who have children.

Alfalfa: Alfalfa is full of nutrition for the entire body. It contains natural fluoride to help strengthen the teeth and prevent tooth decay. It is also used to increase breast milk production in nursing mothers.

Aloe vera: Aloe vera gel can be used externally to soothe and relieve pain on burns, cuts, skin irritations and minor injuries. It is also used to help relieve itching. It helps relieve stomach upset and works as a mild laxative when taken internally.

Barley: This can clean and strengthen the immune system to help fight disease.

Bee Pollen: Bee Pollen can help build the blood and strengthen the body because of its balance of vitamins and minerals. Small doses should be used at first because of possible allergic reactions.

Burdock: Burdock is a great blood purifier to eliminate toxins from the body.

Calendula: This herb contains antiseptic properties and is useful in healing body tissue when suffering from cuts, burns, bruises, or other injuries.

Capsicum (Cayenne): This helps stimulate circulation and the properties of other herbs.

Catnip: This herb can help with colic, gas, indigestion, an upset stomach, and calm the nerves.

Chamomile: This can help settle an upset stomach as well as relax the body. It is often used as a tea and diluted for babies suffering from colic. It can be used to induce sleep and is calming on the nervous system. Some recommend it for teething babies.

Echinacea: Echinacea is a natural antibiotic which helps boost the activity of the immune system. It is often used to treat infections as well as insect bites.

Ephedra (Ma Huang): This has been used successfully in treating sinus congestion, swelling and asthma. It should not be given to children under the age of twelve years unless recommended by a professional. It can cause insomnia and should not be given late in the day.

Fennel: Fennel is used for stomach problems such as colic, indigestion, stomachache and related conditions.

Fenugreek: This is a natural expectorant to help with symptoms of a cold or flu. It can help soothe a sore throat or chest congestion.

Garlic: Although the odor may be unpleasant, garlic is a great natural antibiotic. It is found in some extract formulas as well as odorless capsules. It is helpful for both viral and bacterial infections. It can be used for earaches, respiratory problems, colds, sore throat, fever, and injuries. It can be used as an enema, externally or in liquid or capsule form.

Ginger: This is great for nausea and motion sickness. It can soothe an upset stomach. Ginger is often used to aid in the digestion process. It is also useful for colds and flu, aches and pains, fevers and congestion.

Golden Seal: Golden Seal is a natural antibiotic useful in treating a variety of infections.

Horsetail: Horsetail helps to build the structural system of the body to aid with growth.

Kelp: Kelp contains nutrients valuable for the entire body. It is high in essential minerals.

Licorice: This herb has a pleasant taste. It can help with coughs, colds, flu, and lung congestion. It helps to increase energy in the body. It is also a mild laxative. Caution should be taken with children who suffer from high blood pressure.

Lobelia: It is used for allergies, asthma, bronchitis, croup, and almost all childhood diseases. It aids with relaxation and is thought to help remove obstructions from the body.

Marshmallow: Marshmallow is soothing to the respiratory tract and helpful for sore throats and lung congestion.

Papaya: It aids in the digestive process, and relieves indigestion and gas.

Parsley: Parsley is a natural diuretic which increases urination.

Peppermint: Peppermint is known to strengthen the body. It helps with stomach problems and digestion, as well as heartburn, gas and diarrhea. It can also help reduce fevers.

Red Clover: Red Clover is a blood purifier used to eliminate toxins from the body. It has been used successfully for skin conditions such as acne, rashes, and boils.

Red Raspberry: This can help with colds, colic and fever in children. It is mild and effective in treating childhood illnesses.

Scullcap: Scullcap works as a relaxant on the body. It can help induce sleep and reduce hyperactivity.

Slippery Elm: Slippery Elm is soothing to the digestive tract and is used for constipation, diarrhea, and upset stomach.

Tea Tree Oil: This is helpful in healing infections when applied externally. It can help promote healing and acts as a local anesthetic to relieve pain.

Yellow Dock: Yellow Dock is a mild laxative, detoxifier, and helps with congestion and coughs.

Herbs are available and used in many forms. Some individuals prefer to grow and cultivate their own herbal gardens. Others purchase the herbs in many forms including the following:

Capsules or Tablets: Capsules provide an easy and pleasant method of taking herbs, especially those that are bitter-tasting. They are ground or powdered forms of the herb. When purchased from a well-known and quality company, the herbs can be depended upon to be clean and combined in correct proportions. They are usually prepared and measured by chemists trained in the herb field. Capsules should be taken with a large glass of water or herbal tea to help them dissolve. For children they can be opened and added to yogurt, fruit juice or applesauce.

Compresses: An herbal compress is used to produce similar effects as an ointment but using heat. One or two heaping tablespoons of the herb are boiled in one cup of water. A sterile cotton pad or gauze is dipped in the strained liquid and placed on the affected area while still warm. It can then be covered with a woolen material. Small children should have it bandaged into place. When cold, the compress should be changed. This method is usually used in cases of injury, contusions, and effusions. It is also used when herbs may be too strong to be taken internally and allows them to be absorbed in small amounts.

49

Extracts: Herbal extracts are rubbed into the skin for treating strained muscles and ligaments, arthritis, or inflammation. They can be made with either alcohol or water. They are a concentrated form of the herb, so lesser amounts are needed. They usually contain stimulating herbs such as cayenne and lobelia. Extracts can also be purchased from health food store or professional herb companies.

Ointments: Ointments are used on the skin when the active principles of herbs are needed for extended periods to accelerate healing. They are usually used in cases of injury, contusion and effusion. Some products made from natural sources can be used instead of petroleum products. One or two heaping tablespoons of the herb or herbs are brought to boil in the mixture, which is then stirred or strained. When cold, the ointment is put into jars.

Poultice: A poultice is a warm, mashed, fresh or ground, powdered herb applied directly to the skin to relieve inflammation, blood poisoning, venomous bites, boils, abscess, and to cleanse and heal an affected area. The skin should be oiled before applying the hot poultice. The herb can be mixed with water or another liquid to form a paste. The poultice should be covered with a clean cloth when applied to the affected area.

Salves: Fresh or dried herbs are covered with water, brought to a boil, and simmered for thirty minutes. The herbs are then strained and added to an equal amount of olive or safflower oil. It is simmered until the water has evaporated into steam and only the oil is left. Beeswax can be added to give the mixture a salve consistency. It should be stored in a dark glass jar with a tight lid.

Syrups: Herbs in a syrup base are used for treating coughs, congestion, and throat problems. Syrups are made by adding about two ounces of herbs to a quart of water and gently boiling down to one pint. Honey and or glycerine can be added for flavor. Licorice and wild cherry bark are commonly used as flavorings.

Teas: Herbs can often be made into delicious herbal teas. Many varieties are available at the health food store or even in many grocery stores. Tea is easy for children to take and can be comforting when ill.

Tincture: Tinctures are solutions of concentrated herbal extracts that can be kept for long periods of time. Alcohol is often added as a preservative. Tinctures are useful for herbs that do not taste good or are to be taken over an extended period of time. They may also be used externally as a liniment. Tinctures are generally used with more potent herbs that are usually not used as herbal teas.

IMMUNIZATIONS

Immunizations are intended to give a healthy child a mild or inactivated form of a disease in order to trigger the immune system to develop a resistance to the real disease. More vaccinations are becoming popular and recommended by medical professionals. Some believe them to be helpful and others see them as a source of disease in themselves. As the child is given a small amount of the toxins, the immune system produces antibodies to fight the substance and upon later exposure should be able to produce antibodies to prevent the disease from occurring.

The area of immunizations is certainly controversial. And any parents who have decided not to have their children immunized have felt the wrath of the public school system administrators. What are the controversies involved with immunizing?

There is a growing awareness in the public eye of the dangers associated with immunizations. The trend began years ago with the production of mass immunizations in order to save our children from many of the natural childhood diseases. But the evidence of the benefits of these immunizations are not clear. Some parents opt to take their chances with their children contracting a disease to avoid the risks involved with immunizations.

If a parent chooses not to immunize their child, it is important to make sure the child is fed a healthy diet to avoid the risk of acquiring a disease. They need to ensure the immune system of the child is in optimum condition by providing nutritional, natural food, a calm home and loving environment, and supplements as needed. A parent may choose to have some of the immunizations but not others. They may also decide to begin the course of immunizations after the child is older instead of beginning when they are only two months of age as most pediatricians advise. This gives the child's immune system a chance to mature. Some parents wait until a child is one or two years of age. A child who is not immunized is generally not at risk of acquiring the disease because it would be rare for them to come into contact with an infected individual. And if their immune systems are working properly, the chance would even be less.

One of the major concerns surrounding immunizations is the fact that there have been no long term studies. No one really knows of the subtle damage that may occur in adults immunized as children. Neurological damage, dyslexia, hyperactivity, auto-immune diseases, rheumatoid arthritis, childhood leukemia, AIDS, cancer and lupus are just a few of the conditions some feel are related to immunizations.

It is thought by some that the better living conditions, sanitation, and nutrition in our society today are responsible for the reductions in childhood diseases rather than the immunizations. The long-term effects of the immunizations are really not known. Some have also suggested that diseases go through natural cycles, becoming prevalent at times and then declining for a time. This was seen with polio which was on a decline even before vaccinations. Dr. Robert S. Mendelsohn, M.D. suggests in his book, "There is a growing suspicion that immunization against relatively harmless childhood diseases may be responsible for the dramatic increase in autoimmune diseases since mass inoculations were introduced. These are fearful diseases such as cancer, leukemia, rheumatoid arthritis, multiple sclerosis, Lou Gehrig's disease, lupus erthematosus, and Guillain-Barre syndrome. An autoimmune disease can be explained simply as one in which the body's defense mechanism cannot distinguish between foreign invaders and ordinary body tissues, with the consequence that the body begins to destroy itself. Have we traded mumps and measles for cancer and leukemia?" There are some other disorders that have also been associated with vaccinations such as blood disorders, brain and nervous system diseases, measles, monkey fever, paralysis, SIDS, AIDS, and premature aging.

One concern of many is that the long term effects of immunizations are not fully known. John Gamble says in his book *Vaccination-Exploring Some Myths*, "Most of the infectious diseases are either inhaled or swallowed through the mucous membranes of the lungs and stomach. Here the antigen meets IgA, a particular antibody which lines the mucous membranes. This is the first line of defense. The disease then enters an incubation period of 1-2 weeks before symptoms show; when a vaccine is given, it is injected straight into the bloodstream, avoiding the antibody which lines the mucous membranes. These large amounts of viral genetic tissue and nucleic acid (produced in animal, not human, culture) can, when thus injected, unite with the DNA of human cells. The transformed cells are then recognized by the host's immune system as foreign... These transformed cells, containing latent viruses, may become the focus for the body's own immune system - i.e., the body starts to attack itself."

Many health conscious individuals feel that these childhood diseases are nature's method of eliminating toxins from the body. They regard these diseases as a cleansing process. To not allow the body to use these diseases to cleanse may lead to a suppression of the toxins and to more deadly disease. Most children do fine with these diseases which are relatively mild.

It has been proven that immunizations are not the only factor in determining who will get a particular disease. Nutrition, living conditions, and sanitation are also involved. If a child is healthy and has a strong immune system through proper diet, adequate sleep, and exercise, he will probably only suffer a mild case of a particular disease.

If immunizing is chosen, it would seem beneficial to take measures in building the child's immune system before the vaccination. Vitamin C, Vitamin A, Beta-Carotene, and Acidophilus may all help. Echinacea can also help boost the immune system.

Any vaccination has the potential of adverse reactions. Some of the most common include localized pain, fever, irritability, agitation, and fatigue. Serious ones occur occasionally such as allergic reactions, seizures, blindness, encephalitis, joint pain, brain damage, screaming syndrome and even death. Following immunizations, if serious symptoms occur, seek medical assistance.

Whether to immunize or not is an individual decision. It is important to learn the facts before making that decision. Remember that the child's immune system can be strengthened to help resist disease. This can be achieved by breast feeding and then preparing a nutritious diet for the child.

Common Childhood Vaccinations

*DPT: This is a combination to protect against diphtheria, pertussis and tetanus. Diphtheria is a condition which can be fatal and affects the upper respiratory tract, kidneys, and heart. Pertussis, (whooping cough), can be very dangerous to children under one year of age. Tetanus is an infection that affects the central nervous system.

*DT: This is a combination for diphtheria and tetanus. Complications are more common with the pertussis and some physicians recommend this combination for children at risk.

*Hemophilus Influenzae: This is a meningitis type B vaccine which protects against the common bacterial infection causing meningitis, a potentially fatal condition with serious complications

*Hepatitis B: This protects against hepatitis B that is an infection of the liver and can cause liver disease or even liver cancer.

*MMR: This is a vaccine to prevent against measles, mumps and rubella which, in the past, were fairly common childhood illnesses.

*Polio: This vaccine helps protect against poliomyelitis which can cause paralysis and death. The live vaccine is usually given orally as it is thought of as giving better immunity than the inactivated vaccine. It would not be recommended for a child with a compromised immune system because of the possibility of actually contracting polio.

CHILDHOOD ALLERGIES

An allergy is the body's defense against a substance which is not normally harmful to the body. Pollens, cosmetics, dust, drugs, insect bites and stings, chemicals, foods, molds, and animal hair, to name a few, cannot really hurt the body. They are known as allergens. Just about any substance may cause an allergic reaction in someone, somewhere. The immune system acts to safeguard the body against foreign elements by using the white blood cells to fight them off. When the body wrongly identifies a substance as an invader, the white blood cells can cause symptoms and damage, often causing more harm than the invader. The allergic reaction can become an illness.

There is no clear cut answer as to why some people develop allergies while others do not. Heredity certainly plays a part in the development of allergies. Children of parents with allergies more frequently have allergies. Babies who are not breastfed more often acquire allergies as well. This is why it is important, if possible, to breastfeed the infant. There are many benefits transferred to the child. There also seems to be emotional and stress-related allergy problems. Stress does cause some suppression of the immune system, which may lead to the allergic response.

Stress may not always be emotional. It can come in other ways which attack the body's immune system and destroy its defenses. An onslaught of toxins is stressful, as in the case of sudden exposure to toxic chemicals. This causes an overload on the immune system.

All children come in contact with some form of foreign agents daily. They come in the form of germs, viruses, environmental chemicals, pollutants, pollen, etc. A child under stress is especially vulnerable whether it is physical, emotional, or environmental. This is why it is so important to keep the immune system in top shape.

When the immune system is working well, it can take care of the foreign invaders through the mucous membranes. The sinuses send the allergens down the throat, where they travel to the digestive tract which neutralizes and destroys them. The tonsils, adenoids, and lymphatic system each play an important role in the process of eliminating these harmful substances.

Allergies seem to have increased as industrial technology has developed. Chemicals, pollutants, food additives, herbicides, pesticides, synthetic drugs and processed foods may have added to this rise.

There are many problems that some doctors have linked to childhood allergies. Some include:.

BEDWETTING

Nocturnal Enuresis commonly called bedwetting which persists beyond the age of three may be linked to allergies. Some believe the major allergens affecting this problem are milk and milk products, wheat, eggs, corn, chocolate, and pork. Inhalants such as pollens, house dust, molds, and animal hair may also cause bedwetting. The problems seems to be in the decreased bladder capacities due to allergies. Fluid builds up in the layers of the bladder and cause it to swell. When the allergen is removed, the bladder will most likely return to normal size.

HYPERACTIVITY

Allergies may also be linked to hyperkinetic activity in children. The most common offenders include milk, wheat, eggs, chocolate, sugar and food dyes. Some children can't sit still, concentrate, control emotions, and sleep. This may be due to allergies which cause them to feel out of control and unable to sit for any amount of time.

RESPIRATORY

The respiratory system is often linked to allergies. Many think of sniffles, itchy eyes and a cough when they think of allergies. This type of allergic response is often caused by milk and wheat products, as well as pollens and pollutants in the air. Some allergy symptoms include asthma, coughs, colds, hay fever, sinusitis, nose bleeds, wheezing, shortness of breath, and tightness in the chest.

CEREBRAL

It has just been in recent years that cerebral or brain allergies have been recognized. These may show up in the form of schizophrenia, depression, hallucinations, delusions, catatonia, etc. These symptoms are caused by a swelling of the lining of the brain. Many patients have been helped with these problems through controlling allergies. Many different substances, among them auto exhaust, corn, plastic, environmental toxins, etc., may trigger symptoms in sensitive individuals. Some other manifestations of cerebral allergies include anxiety, dizzy spells, nervousness, insomnia, learning disorders, restlessness, and fatigue.

GASTROINTESTINAL

Gastrointestinal allergies often accompany respiratory allergies in a majority of cases. These allergies have the same symptoms as ailments such as ulcers, colitis, appendicitis, heartburn, indigestion, nausea, diarrhea, constipation, and intestinal gas.

CARDIOVASCULAR

Allergies can affect the cardiovascular system. When an allergen is introduced into the body allergic symptoms may include hypertension, rapid pulse, high or low blood pressure, or irregular heartbeat.

SKIN

Skin problems have been linked to allergic responses. Some types of allergies may be caused by a toxic colon or contact with detergents or other topical substances to which a person is sensitive. Some symptoms include acne, blisters, blotches, flushing, dark circles under the eyes, eczema, hives, itching, and psoriasis.

NERVOUS SYSTEM

Allergic responses by the nervous system can be caused by many different factors, including poisonous substances, foods, chemicals or preservatives. These are often linked with cerebral allergies and symptoms include migraines, drowsiness, depression, anger, anxiety, irritability, restlessness, and lack of concentration. Some health professionals feel that Attention Deficit Disorder (ADD) and other problems dealing with concentration may be linked to allergies.

EAR

These manifestations of allergies are often linked to respiratory allergies. Children who often suffer from ear infections may have allergy problems. Most common allergens are wheat, sugar, milk, chocolate, pollens and other inhaled allergens. Some symptoms are frequent ear infections, itching in ears, dizziness, imbalance, sensitivity to noise, and earaches.

HEALTHY SLEEP PATTERNS

Putting a baby to bed can be one of the most frustrating experiences imaginable. The new parent is not accustomed to being awakened two, three, four, or more times during the night. A lack of sleep can cause both parent and child to be irritable, upset, and more susceptible to illness. Sleep is essential, and developing good sleep habits should begin from the start.

There is a wide variation in sleep patterns of newborns as well as all children. But a lack of sleep can result in a problems for all concerned. A child not getting enough sleep may be listless, drowsy or hyperactive. Marc Weissbluth, M.D. in his book *Healthy Sleep Habits, Happy Child* on page 6 states, "Sleep problems not only disrupt a child's nights, they disrupt his days too, (a) by making him less mentally alert, more inattentive, unable to concentrate, or easily distracted, and (b) by making him more physically impulsive, hyperactive, or alternatively lazy. But when our children sleep well, they are optimally awake and optimally alert to learn and to grow up with charm, humor, and love. When parents are too irregular, inconsistent, or over solicitous, when mothers or fathers are overly absorbed in their children, when marital problems are left unresolved, the resulting sleep problems converge in the final condition: excessive nighttime wakefulness and crying"

Parents can help set good sleep patterns for their children. Regular nap times and regular bed times are important. This may exclude the child or adult from some activities until a healthy sleep pattern is developed. Keeping a child up past their natural bedtime can be detrimental. A child who is sleepy and ready for bed but kept awake may exhaust his nervous system. This can result in hyperactivity and sleeplessness when the child is finally put to bed. A regular routine can solve the problem with firmness when needed.

Napping will vary in children. Some will continue napping until they are four or even five. But some will rebel beginning at the age of two. If the nap is discontinued, remember an earlier bedtime may be necessary. Adjust schedules as necessary to ensure adequate sleep.

Bedtime should be a pleasant time. Stories, songs or cuddling before bed can bring pleasant, peaceful feelings. Avoid giving too much food to the child before bed. Some children may ask for food when they are tired. Plan calm and quiet activities before the child goes to bed. This can help them relax before bed. Try and make bedtime a good time.

ANTIBIOTICS

Some medical professionals would have you believe that the only way to cure some ailments is through antibiotic therapy. But before the discovery of antibiotics, ear infections and tonsillitis were often cured even though there were some who did develop severe problems. Antibiotics have taken on a new light in recent years. Fifteen years ago, antibiotics were prescribed routinely when a fever was present by some pediatricians. But with the onset of drug resistant strains of bacteria, more health practitioners are realizing their mistakes. Now antibiotics are usually saved for severe conditions as a last resort. Most agree that antibiotics are useful for killing large amounts of bacteria. But the good bacteria are also destroyed.

Antibiotics should not be used without looking into the cause. The body contains its own defense system. The immune system is powerful. It is a good idea to use means to ensure the strength of the immune system.

Ear infections are often treated routinely with antibiotics. Dr. Mendelsohn said in his book *How To Raise A Healthy Child...In Spite Of Your Doctor* on pages 130-131, "As the years passed I learned that many of my patients, perhaps the majority, failed to take their antibiotics for the time period prescribed, and many of them never got the prescription filled at all. In medical circles this kind of behavior is called 'patient noncompliance,' and it is frowned upon by doctors and pharmaceutical manufacturers alike. But what disturbed me more than noncompliance was the realization that my noncompliant patients recovered from their infections as rapidly as those who complied, and not one of them ever went deaf!

"At first I consoled myself by invoking the standard line that all doctors are taught to recite when their patients get well by ignoring their advised: 'You're lucky, that's all.' Before long that rationalization no longer satisfied me, because so many untreated patients had recovered without medication that there couldn't be that much luck to go around."

"That destroyed my faith in antibiotics, and I quit prescribing them, with no apparent negative effect on my patients."

If antibiotics are necessary, be sure and give extra vitamins and herbal supplements to help the immune system. Acidophilus is necessary to help restore the normal intestinal bacteria lost during the antibiotic course.

PART II
COMMON CHILDHOOD AILMENTS

ACNE

Acne is most commonly seen in adolescents but may begin in childhood and continue into adulthood. It affects approximately eighty percent of the population to some degree. Lesions may appear around puberty, and most children suffer from some degree of acne. It is a condition involving inflammation of the skin in the form of pimples, blackheads and whiteheads. The sebaceous glands produce oils which moisturize the skin. These glands increase in number at the onset of puberty when hormonal changes occur in the body. When the oils are blocked from exiting the skin surface, irritations occur causing the acne. There may also be an increase in bacteria normally found in the glands. When a blockage occurs, inflammation may result, causing a pimple.

Babies often get a form of acne around four to six weeks of age. It is common and caused by the hormone adjustment of the baby. It does not require treatment and usually lasts just a few weeks.

Chronic acne can be a serious problem for many adolescents. At a time in life when appearance is extremely important and peer pressure is strong, acne can cause withdrawal and depression. Emotionally, acne can be very difficult. Natural methods are necessary to treat the cause of the problem.

CAUSES

The reason for acne is often not understood. The sebaceous glands are located in the hair follicles beneath the skin. They produce the oil that helps to moisten and lubricate the skin. When the oil is clogged in the gland, bacteria can multiply and cause inflammation or even infection. Hormonal changes may be a factor in susceptible individuals. Poor hygiene can worsen the condition when the skin surface is not kept clean. Ingredients in some cosmetics and moisturizers, such as mineral oil or petroleum-based ingredients, can cause the pores to clog and aggravate the condition. Some substances thought to cause acne include ammonia, formaldehyde, artificial colors, nitrates, and artificial fragrances. Drugs such as steroids, birth control pills, phenothiazine, Dilantin, lithium, and iodides have been linked to outbreaks of acne. Heredity may also contribute to the acne.

Originally, diet was not considered a factor in acne. But now some dermatologists and acne sufferers see a connection between certain foods and acne. Foods thought to cause problems include fatty foods, fried foods, chocolate, nuts, sweets, and sugar. Allergies to certain foods may also be a problem. Some cases of acne may be attributed to poor fat metabolism. Foods that contain hormones such as beef, chicken, dairy products and eggs, may cause hormone imbalances which may contribute to acne.

Stress can also be a factor in acne. Stress causes the release of higher levels of certain hormones. This causes an increase in the production of sebum which can lead to clogged pores. Stress lowers the body's immune response, which can aggravate the problem.

Many natural health practitioners see constipation as a contributing factor to acne. The kidneys and liver help to clean the blood. When the colon is congested or constipation is a problem, the toxins may back up in the kidneys and liver and be excreted through the skin. This can be a factor in developing acne.

HOME CARE

- Keep the skin as clean as possible. Use a mild soap, such as castile soap, and wash twice a day.
- Use a warm wash cloth to help clean the pores.
- Apply a compress of papaya mint tea. Steep two tea bags in 3/4 cup boiling water. Cool to warm and apply a compress.
- Mild exposure to the sun can help the skin. This should be avoided if on medication for acne. Check with your health care professional.
- Applying a clay pack to the skin will help draw out the toxins.
- Lemon juice can be dabbed on the affected areas of the skin. Avoid the eye area.

DIETARY GUIDELINES

- As constipation may contribute to the problem, eating a diet high in fiber can help keep the colon functioning properly. A fiber supplement may be useful.
- Increase the intake of fresh fruits and vegetables. Eating these raw will ensure the consumption of enzymes, vitamins and minerals.
- Drink plenty of bottled spring water to help rid the body of toxins.
- Eat a well-balanced diet high in fruits, vegetables, and whole grains. Eat natural foods which are free of additives and preservatives which may contribute to acne outbreaks.

- Decrease fat in the diet. Limit animal fat and hydrogenated oils.
- Juices such as carrot, celery, and citrus fruit juices are beneficial.
- Cherries and grapes naturally cleanse toxins from the blood.
- Avoid foods such as alcohol, chocolate, fatty foods, fried foods, and sugar.

NUTRITIONAL SUPPLEMENTS

- **Vitamin C with Bioflavonoids:** This can help enhance the function of the immune system to help prevent and clear up acne. Vitamin C is known to improve connective tissue health and the bioflavonoids help with inflammation.
- **B-Complex Vitamins:** Stress is a contributing factor in some cases of acne. The B vitamins are known to help the body handle stress. They contribute to healthy skin and in fighting infection.
- **Vitamin E:** This is known to help prevent scarring. It helps regulate the balance of vitamin A in the body. Selenium in combination with vitamin E can also help promote healthy skin.
- **Vitamin A and Beta-Carotene:** Vitamin A and Beta-carotene are both healing for the skin. They can strengthen the epithelial layer of the skin. They also help in boosting the immune system.
- **Calcium and Magnesium:** This can help strengthen the nervous system and may decrease the desire for sugar that can contribute to acne problems.
- **Zinc:** Zinc is beneficial for tissue growth and healing. It also helps with the development of the reproductive system. It aids in reducing inflammation and in healing the skin and mucous membranes.

- **Chromium:** Chromium is known to help balance blood sugar levels. It aids in reducing inflammations of the skin.
- **Niacin:** Niacin helps increase blood circulation to the skin.
- **Acidophilus:** Acidophilus helps increase the friendly bacteria in the intestines. It can also help with constipation which may contribute to acne problems. It is especially important when antibiotics are taken.
- **Chlorophyll/Blue-Green Algae:** These can help purify the blood and clear toxins from the body.
- **Indoles:** Dietary indoles, found in some supplements, can help strengthen the immune system and aid in skin health.

HERBAL REMEDIES

- **Alfalfa:** Alfalfa helps fight infection, strengthen the immune system, and clear toxins from the body.
- **Red Clover:** This can help cleanse the blood of toxins.
- **Garlic:** Garlic contains healing properties and also helps strengthen the immune system and promote sweating.
- **Lavender:** Lavender can help in killing germs and bacteria and to encourage the growth of new cells.
- **Golden Seal:** Golden Seal contains anti-bacterial properties, fights infection and helps clear toxins from the body.
- **Echinacea:** It helps strengthen the immune system to prevent illness and infection.
- **Oregon Grape:** It has been used for skin ailments.
- **Aloe Vera:** Aloe Vera is great for any skin disorder. It is healing, refreshing and helps prevent scarring. Supplements can be taken internally or the gel can be applied directly to the skin.
- **Tea Tree Oil:** Diluted Tea Tree Oil can be applied to the skin to help heal and prevent infection, as it contains anti-bacterial properties and will promote healing.

- **Psyllium:** Increased fiber can help reduce constipation which may contribute to cases of acne.
- **Yellow Dock:** It helps to purify the blood and heal infection due to antibiotic properties.
- **Burdock:** Burdock can help to promote sweating to clear toxins through the skin. It also helps to purify the blood.
- **Herbal combinations** can also be beneficial to clean the blood and fight infection. Combinations to purify the blood and improve bowel function could help.

ALLERGIES
(Also see section on Childhood Allergies)

Allergy symptoms are triggered when the body reacts to substances that are not normally harmful. There are many different substances when eaten, inhaled or come into contact with the skin's surface that may trigger an allergic response. Some common substances which may bring on an allergic reaction include pollens, cosmetics, dust, drugs, insect bites and stings, chemicals, foods, milk, wheat, seafood, nuts, molds, and animal hair. Just about anything may cause an allergic reaction in a susceptible individual. The immune system acts to safeguard the body against foreign bodies by using the white blood cells to fight them off. When the body identifies a substance as an invader, the white blood cells cause symptoms and maybe even damage. An allergy may be an over reaction of the immune system which uses antibodies to attack the foreign invader. The antibodies produce histamine and serotonin which cause inflammation resulting in a runny nose, sneezing, itching, watery eyes, etc. The allergic reaction can become an illness.

CAUSES

Allergies do not affect everyone. There are really no clear cut answer as to why some people develop allergies. Heredity seems to be part of the reason for the development of allergies. Children of parents with allergies more frequently have allergies. Breast feeding seems to offer an advantage over bottle feeding in the prevention of allergies. Some of the mother's antibodies are transferred to the child which give added protection. During the first few months of a baby's life, their intestines and lung membranes are not fully developed. This can cause problems as particles enter the body causing the production of antibodies. According to Thomas J. Young in an article in *Let's Live*, August 1990, the elevated levels of IgE antibodies are associated with conditions such as eczema, inflammation and allergies. This is another reason that breast feeding can be beneficial. There also seems to be emotional and stress related allergy problems. Stress does cause some suppression of the immune system which may lead to the allergic response. Stress may not always be emotional. It can come in other ways which attack the body's immune system and destroy its defenses. An onslaught of toxins is stressful, as in the case of sudden exposure to toxic chemicals. This causes an overload on the immune system. Children are exposed to toxins daily. A child may be under stress whether due to physical, emotional, or environmental factors.

If the immune system is working well, it can take care of the foreign invaders through the mucous membranes. The sinuses send the allergens down the throat where they travel to the digestive tract which neutralizes and destroys them. The tonsils, adenoids, and lymphatic system each play an important role in the process of eliminating these harmful substances.

Some allergies to foods may occur when a child eats the same food all the time. The body may develop a reaction after continuous exposure. Eating a variety of foods can help. To verify a food allergy, eat one food at a time. Take the pulse before eating the food and then twenty minutes after. If the pulse is rapid, this may indicate an allergic response. Poor digestion may contribute to toxic buildup which can contribute to allergies.

Allergies seem to have increased as industrial technology has increased. Chemicals, pollutants, food additives, herbicides, pesticides, synthetic drugs and processed foods may have added to this rise. The overuse of antibiotics such as penicillin may be a factor in allergies.

HOME CARE

- Use a warm saline solution as a nasal spray.
- Replace furnace filters often to keep the dust down.
- Wash stuffed toys, blankets and rugs often, as they collect dust mites which are common allergens.
- Avoid known allergens as much as possible.

DIETARY GUIDELINES

- Avoid substances that bring on an allergic reaction.
- Avoid foods such as wheat, eggs, dairy products, chocolate, nuts, caffeine, shellfish, strawberries, tomatoes, and citrus fruits. These are commonly associated with food allergies.
- Avoid additives in foods such as preservatives and pesticides.
- Brown rice is a great food full of nutritional value.
- Fruits containing pits such as cherries and peaches aid in elimination and are non-allergenic. Peel the peaches before giving them to children as the peach fuzz may cause allergic reactions.

- Add fiber to the diet to keep the bowels functioning effectively. Some nutritionists believe that constipation is a leading cause of allergy problems.
- Raw honey contains pollen that may help in building a resistance to hay fever. Introduce slowly to the diet and watch for allergic reactions.
- Rita Elkins in her book, *The Complete Home Health Advisor*, suggests brewer's yeast, grapefruit, and wheat germ blended together in a drink to help build the cell walls and to increase immune function. The brewer's yeast should not be used if there is a sensitivity to yeast products.

NUTRITIONAL SUPPLEMENTS

- **Vitamin A:** It helps heal and soothe the mucous membranes. It is an antioxidant to help build the immune function which can prevent allergies.
- **B-Complex Vitamins:** The B-complex vitamins are also helpful for the membranes, reducing stress, and aiding in the digestion process.
- **Vitamin C and Bioflavonoids:** Vitamin C with bioflavonoids help with adrenal and immune function and aids in protecting against allergies. They work as antioxidants to prevent free radical damage and protect the immune system.
- **Minerals:** A multi-mineral supplement will help protect against the toxic effects of heavy metals. Minerals are essential to health and for all body functions.
- **Calcium/Magnesium:** Calcium and magnesium help protect against infections. Magnesium may help individuals suffering from allergy-related asthma.
- **Potassium:** Potassium helps with neuromuscular impulses.

- **Acidophilus:** Acidophilus aids in the digestion process and helps eliminate undigested protein.
- **Blue-Green Algae/Chlorophyll:** Blue-green algae cleans the blood and nourishes the mucous membranes.
- **Tyrosine:** Tyrosine is an amino acid which helps with allergies hay fever related from grass pollens.
- **Essential Fatty Acids:** The essential fatty acids help with digestion and assimilation. They are often lacking in children's diets.

HERBAL REMEDIES

- **Angelica:** Angelica helps with the formation of antibodies.
- **Bee Pollen:** Bee Pollen has been used successfully as a gradual method of building immunity. A small amount should be used initially, gradually adding a little more at a time while watching for allergic reactions. Many have been treated successfully using Bee Pollen.
- **Burdock:** Burdock works as a blood purifier to clean toxins from the body.
- **Echinacea:** Echinacea is a natural antibiotic and immune builder. It can be given to children in an extract form.
- **Garlic:** Garlic is another natural antibiotic to help fight infection and strengthen the immune system.
- **Licorice:** Licorice helps strengthen and soothe the mucous membranes. It contains anti-inflammatory and anti-allergic properties.
- **Lobelia:** Lobelia is wonderful for loosening obstructions in the body. It can work to remove bronchial congestion and spasms. It is a natural relaxant.
- **Ma Huang:** Ma Huang (Ephedra) is an antihistamine and has been found effective for treating conditions such as asthma, allergies, and bronchitis. Caution should be used in children under the age of twelve years. Check with a health practitioner.

- **Ginger:** Ginger helps with digestion and assimilation of foods.
- **Golden Seal:** Golden Seal has natural antibiotic and healing properties.
- **Milk Thistle:** This helps to clean the liver and improve the liver function which may be impaired when allergies are a problem.
- **Herbal combinations** to strengthen the liver, improve bowel function, and purify the blood could be helpful.

ANEMIA

Anemia is a condition that can have many different symptoms. Some of them include depression, fainting, fatigue, headaches, indigestion, irritability, immune disorders, frequent colds and infections, angina pectoris, poor coloring, and general weakness. Anemia can easily be detected through a blood test.

Anemia is considered to be a lack of hemoglobin in the blood. Iron is found in the heme of hemoglobin. In the spleen, bone marrow and liver it is known as ferritin and hemosiderin. Iron is lost each day in secretions of the body and must be replaced by food or supplements. Iron is concentrated in the red blood cells which are made in the bone marrow. The red blood cells carry oxygen to all parts of the body. The amount of oxygen that the blood can carry is reduced.

There are many different types of anemia, the most common being associated with an iron deficiency. This is important because iron is essential in the production of hemoglobin which carries oxygen. There is usually a deficiency of folic acid and vitamin B12 as well. Sickle-cell anemia, most commonly found in the African-American population, is another condition of anemia.

Infants and children not eating well may be susceptible to anemia. Even though infant formulas contain iron supplements, anemia is still a possibility. The iron is hard for the body to absorb. Children should be fed a variety of foods and a supplement when necessary. Another factor may be failure to absorb the nutrients available. Phyllis Austin, Agatha Thrash M.D. and Calvin Thrash, M.D. M.P.H. in their book *Natural Healthcare For Your Child*, on page 25 say "Peak incidence of iron deficiency anemia occurs in the six-month to two-year old group, then declines to rise again during adolescence. Adolescent females are more likely to become iron deficient than males because of iron loss associated with menstrual periods."

CAUSES

Anemia can be caused by excessive bleeding and malnutrition. Children who are allergic to cow's milk are susceptible to anemia. An allergic reaction may result in gastrointestinal bleeding which may cause small amounts of blood to be lost over a long period of time, resulting in anemia. And children who drink a lot of milk may not be eating enough iron rich foods which also leads to anemia. This is quite common in children and is referred to as "milk anemia." Children need to be able to utilize the iron made available to them. If it isn't absorbed, it won't help the problem. Other factors which may contribute to anemia include infection, surgery, ulcers, hormonal disorders, liver disorders, thyroid problems, excessive menstrual flow, and poor nutrition.

HOME CARE

- Mild sun exposure daily can help stimulate the production of red blood cells.
- When taking a supplement, increase fiber and liquid intake to avoid constipation.

DIETARY GUIDELINES

- Breast feeding for a year helps prevent anemia.
- Milk should be eliminated from the diet as a possible cause of the problem.
- Refined foods should be restricted.
- Foods rich in iron should be eaten such as green leafy vegetables, wheat germ, cherries, grape juice, bananas, raisins, prunes, whole grain breads, dried apricots, blackstrap molasses, raw egg yolks, dried beans and peas, soy beans and prune juice.
- Foods to avoid are those with oxalic acid which interferes with the absorption of iron. Some include almonds, chocolate, kale, soda, and nuts. Additives found in some foods such as beer, dairy products, ice cream, and candy bars as well as tea and coffee also interfere.
- Whole and natural foods are important for better nutrient absorption.
- Vitamin C aids in the absorption of iron. Eat vitamin C rich foods.
- Vegetables, legumes, grains and seeds can help with iron absorption.
- Black strap molasses is high in iron and B-vitamins.

NUTRITIONAL SUPPLEMENTS

- **Iron:** A natural iron supplement may be advised. Liquid formulas are often prescribed for children. Take between meals for better absorption. This may cause stomach upset. Adding iron rich foods to the diet is preferable.
- **Vitamin C and Bioflavonoids:** Vitamin C with bioflavonoids aid in the absorption of iron. If taking a supplement of iron, take C at the same time.
- **B-Complex:** B vitamins help in the assimilation of food.
- **Multi-Minerals:** A multi-mineral supplement is essential.
- **Chlorophyll/Blue-Green Algae:** These are rich in iron and help build the blood.
- **Copper, Manganese, Cobalt, and Magnesium:** These are all necessary for hemoglobin formation.

HERBAL REMEDIES

- **Alfalfa:** Alfalfa is very nutritious and rich in minerals.
- **Burdock:** This herb is a great blood purifier. It contains high amounts of vitamin C and iron.
- **Kelp:** Kelp is rich in essential minerals easily absorbed by the body.
- **Red Raspberry:** This herb is rich in iron and other essential vitamins and minerals. It can be given in a tea form safely for both infants and children.
- **Slippery Elm:** Slippery Elm aids in the digestion and absorption of nutrients. It is rich in essential vitamins and minerals.
- **Garlic:** Garlic may help in cases of anemia.
- **Yellow Dock:** Yellow Dock is rich in organic iron easily assimilated in the body.
- **Dandelion:** This helps the liver to absorb the iron.
- **Comfrey:** Comfrey is useful for treating anemia.

APPENDICITIS

Appendicitis is an acute inflammation of the appendix which is a thin, oblong protrusion off of the large intestine. It is a worm shaped appendage that is attached to the cecum, the first part of the large intestine. The inflammation can be caused by hardened fecal matter blocking the intestine or a structural problem. This condition can easily lead to infection causing serious problems.

A child may complain of pain in the stomach, moving to the lower right side of the abdomen. A child will probably lose his appetite, vomit, have a fever, and react when pressure is applied lightly to the area. It can be extremely painful and may require immediate medical attention.

The major concern is that the appendix may burst, spreading the infection throughout the abdominal area. A continuous pain in the stomach area should be taken seriously and medical attention is recommended.

CAUSES

Appendicitis is usually a gradually occurring condition. It is thought that constipation is a leading cause of appendicitis. Obstructions of the intestines can result in improper drainage. A diet low in fiber is a contributing factor.

HOME CARE

• The child should get plenty of rest after an appendicitis attack or surgery in order for the body to fully recover.
• Avoid too much activity for up to six weeks following surgery.
• To avoid the problem, keep the immune system functioning well, include fiber in the diet, and eat natural

wholesome foods.
- Removing the appendix may cause the bowel to become sensitive and lead to constipation. Remember to include fiber rich foods, prune juice and a lot of pure water in the diet.

DIETARY GUIDELINES

- Add food gradually after an attack or surgery, beginning with liquids such as broth, juices, and herbal teas.
- A juice fast for a few days may help healing. Beet juice, carrot juice and grape juice are all beneficial.
- Applesauce, fruit juice and homemade vegetable soups are easy to digest after appendix surgery.
- Eat a diet rich in fiber foods.
- Whole grains, baked potatoes (with skins), brown rice, beans, sprouts, fresh and steamed vegetables, and fruit are all nutritious and beneficial.
- Avoid gas producing foods at first, such as nuts and beans.
- Prune juice can help the bowels function properly.

NUTRITIONAL SUPPLEMENTS

- **Beta-Carotene/Vitamin A:** Beta-carotene and vitamin A can help soothe and heal the mucous membranes and damaged tissue.
- **B-Complex:** The B-complex vitamins help promote healing and strength.
- **Vitamin C and Bioflavonoids:** Vitamin C along with bioflavonoids are healing and help with inflammation.
- **Vitamin E:** Vitamin E is healing to the tissues and an antioxidant to strengthen the immune system.
- **Zinc:** Zinc is known to help aid in wound healing and to strengthen the immune system.

- **Multi-Mineral:** A multi-mineral supplement is helpful in strengthening the body and nourishing the blood.
- **Chlorophyll/Blue-Green Algae:** These are healing and help clear toxins from the body.

HERBAL REMEDIES

- **Aloe Vera:** Aloe Vera is healing and soothing on the intestinal tract.
- **Echinacea:** Echinacea helps with healing and to prevent infection with or without surgery. It will help immune function.
- **Garlic:** Garlic is also helpful in preventing or healing infection.
- **Golden Seal:** Golden Seal is an immune builder as well as an aid in healing and preventing infection.
- **Kelp:** Kelp is high in minerals which are healing to the body.
- **Passion Flower:** Passion Flower helps with inflammation, pain and relaxes and calms the nervous system. It contains anti-inflammatory properties.
- **Slippery Elm:** Slippery Elm is healing to the intestinal tract. It can help soothe and heal internal wounds.
- **Cascara Sagrada:** This will help with constipation to avoid the problem and as a laxative after surgery or an inflammation.
- **Catnip:** This can be used as an enema to promote healing.
- **A nervine herb combination** can help calm the nerves and relax the body for healing.

ASTHMA

Asthma is an inflammatory condition of the respiratory tract, causing mild or severe difficulty in breathing. The airways of the lungs constrict making breathing labored. The muscles involved with breathing spasm, narrowing the airway tubes. Excess mucus can also cause the smaller tubes to clog and constrict. Attacks can vary in length from a few minutes to a week in length, with periodic spasms. Asthma is a condition of the respiratory tract with recurrent attacks of constrained breathing, tight chest and wheezing when exhaling. The two main types of asthma include extrinsic in which the attack is an allergic response and intrinsic in which there is no apparent external cause.

Asthma can occur in children but not usually until the age of three. Over half of the children who have asthma will outgrow the condition as they grow older, and the incidence of asthma is higher in boys than girls. Asthma attacks often occur when a child is nervous or tense. Anxiety can bring on an attack. A child with this condition will put a lot of effort into breathing and this can cause abnormal breathing patterns because of the tense state in which the abdomen muscles remain even after an attack subsides. The nerves associated with breathing have connections to the nerves which are associated with spasms in the lungs.

CAUSES

Asthma is often associated with allergies and can be triggered by allergens such as dust, pollen, cigarette smoke, molds, animal hair, foods, etc. The allergen causes a constriction of the bronchiole tubes, located within the lungs, resulting in breathing difficulty. Asthma may also occur after a respiratory infection, cold, sinus condition, or other respiratory problems. Recent studies have found that asthma can be brought on by exercising in cold conditions. Some athletes, having never experienced breathing difficulties, developed asthma after running and breathing cold air. Asthma is quite common among athletes, especially runners.

Heredity does seem to be a factor in those who develop asthma. Children of parents with asthma are more likely to acquire asthma. But the exact cause of the condition is not known. The reason that the nerves cause the bronchiole tubes to constrict is not fully understood.

Cases of asthma continue to increase. Many believe the reason for the rise in incidences of asthma are due to air pollution, pollution in homes, toxins, poor diet, free radical damage and chemical additives. Constipation may also be a factor in cases of asthma because of the toxins accumulating in the body. Stress can also contribute to asthma. Emotions seem to be linked to asthma attacks.

HOME CARE

- Keep children away from smoke filled rooms even if they are not prone to lung problems. Children of smokers have a greater risk of developing asthma as well as other lung related problems.
- If taking medication, follow directions carefully.
- Exercise helps improve the lung function.
- Help the child learn to relax and to use deep breathing techniques.
- Avoid sudden exposure to cold air.
- Drink pure water to dilute mucus secretions.
- Chiropractic treatments may help normalize nerve action by releasing nerve pressure.
- Avoid food additives such as BHA and BHT, and food colorings.

DIETARY GUIDELINES

- Avoid milk and milk products. The proteins in milk products may cause excess mucus secretions.
- A healthy, whole-food diet should be used. Use whole grains, brown rice, oatmeal, seeds, nuts, lean proteins, fruits and vegetables in the diet.
- Make sure there is a lot of fiber in the diet to ensure adequate bowel function.
- Avoid foods which may cause allergic reactions such as nuts, wheat, milk, seafood, additives, etc. White flour products should also be avoided.
- Drink a lot of pure water.
- A glass of pure water with fresh lemon or lime juice can help with asthma.
- Avoid cold drinks and foods such as ice cream which may stimulate an attack.

NUTRITIONAL SUPPLEMENTS

- **Magnesium:** According to some research, magnesium levels may be low in asthmatics. Adequate amounts of magnesium may help prevent bronchial spasms and have a bronchial dilating effect. Bronchial spasms may result in excess mucus.
- **Calcium:** Calcium is essential to nerve impulse transmission.
- **Beta-Carotene:** This is essential for healing and the mucous membranes. It has been found to help protect the lungs in children and to strengthen the immune system.
- **Vitamin C and Bioflavonoids:** Vitamin C can help with allergies and asthma. It may also help reduce the severity of asthma in children. It is a natural anti-inflammatory and helps strengthen the connective tissue. The bioflavonoid quercetin may help inhibit histamine production and

prevent the release of chemical leukotrienes which cause spasms of the bronchioles.

- **Vitamin A:** This helps build immunity and promotes the healing process.
- **Vitamin E:** Vitamin E is an anti-oxidant vitamin and helps strengthen the immune system as well as helping heal tissue and reduce scarring.
- **Essential Fatty Acids:** Essential fatty acids are important in preventing inflammation. They increase the oxygen carrying capacity of the blood. They may be lacking in a child's diet and should be supplemented if necessary.
- **B-Complex Vitamins:** The B-complex vitamins work together, and when giving a single B vitamin, a B-complex should be taken as well.
- **Vitamin B5 (Pantothenic Acid):** Vitamin B5 is important for the nervous system and adrenal action.
- **Vitamin B6:** This vitamin has been found to help in reducing the severity of asthma attacks.
- **Vitamin B12:** This has been shown to help children in treating asthma especially with wheezing. It is also used to boost the immune system and reduce stress.
- **Selenium:** It helps in protecting the immune system and in strengthening the cardiovascular system.
- **Zinc:** Zinc helps the immune system and in healing.
- **Indoles:** Dietary indoles can help strengthen the immune system.

HERBAL REMEDIES

- **Astragalus:** Astragalus is a Chinese herb used to increase the protective energy in the body and to strengthen the lungs. This herb should not be used in cases where infection or fever are present.
- **Comfrey:** This herb is effective on the respiratory system. It helps reduce mucus and congestion.

- **Ephedra:** This herb has been used for thousands of years in treating asthma. It is useful in reducing congestion and as a bronchiodilator. It should be avoided in children under twelve years.
- **Fenugreek:** Fenugreek works as an expectorant in removing mucus and helps in fighting infection.
- **Garlic:** Garlic is a natural antibiotic. It helps the formation of antibodies in the immune system. It also helps with lung congestion.
- **Ginger:** Ginger contains some natural antibiotic properties to inhibit the growth of bacteria. It can help with respiratory problems.
- **Golden Seal:** Golden Seal works as a natural antibiotic. It is healing and strengthening to the immune system.
- **Licorice:** Licorice helps in soothing the lungs and to help adrenal function. It contains anti-inflammatory and anti-allergenic properties similar to the corticosteroid drugs. It should be used with caution for children suffering from blood sugar problems.
- **Lobelia:** This herb helps to clear obstructions from the body. It is a powerful relaxant and anti-spasmodic.
- **Marshmallow:** Marshmallow helps soothe the bronchial tubes.
- **Mullein:** Mullein acts as a bronchial decongestant and is known to help prevent as well as lessen the severity of asthma attacks. It contains antispasmodic properties useful for asthmatics.
- **Slippery Elm:** Slippery Elm is healing to the mucous membranes of the body.
- **Thyme:** Thyme contains antispasmodic and antibacterial properties to help heal and prevent asthma spasms. Steam inhalation with thyme can help open up the bronchial tubes.

ATHLETE'S FOOT

Athlete's foot is a fungus that can be annoying and persistent. It is a common skin condition found in children and adults whether they are athletes or not. It is probably the most common fungal infection which thrives in a moist, warm environment and is often found in athletic shoes, sweaty socks, gyms and pool areas. It is a contagious condition, and some individuals seem to be more susceptible. It is characterized by itching, burning, scaling and tiny blisters between the toes and on the bottom of the feet.

Keeping the feet clean and dry can help prevent athlete's foot. Air the feet out as much as possible. Wash socks in hot water to kill the fungus and keep it from spreading. Wash the feet in soap and water and wear white, cotton socks, if possible, to allow the feet to breathe.

CAUSES

Athlete's foot is caused by a fungus similar to ringworm known as dermatophyte. It occurs when an individual spends long periods of time in moist socks and shoes. It can be passed from individual to individual in locker rooms and showers. The condition of the immune system may play a role in those who are susceptible to athlete's foot. Antibiotics and a high sugar diet may contribute, as the good bacteria may be destroyed allowing for the fungal growth. Skin conditions may be related to congestion in the colon and kidneys.

HOME CARE

- Expose feet to the air as often as possible to allow them to dry out.
- Wash the feet with soap and water at least twice daily. Dry

the feet carefully and dry between toes.
- Wear slippers or thongs in public locker rooms and pool areas.
- Wash socks in chlorine bleach to stop the condition from spreading.
- Avoid scratching, as infection may occur.
- A baking soda paste can help ease the itching.
- Soak the feet in warm salt water for five to ten minutes. (2 t. salt to 1 pint water)
- Wear white cotton socks to allow the feet to breathe.
- Soak the feet in water and vinegar to help kill the fungus.

DIETARY GUIDELINES

- Eliminate sugar from the diet. Soda and processed foods contain high amounts of sugar. The sugar encourages the growth of fungus.
- Have the child eat a wholesome diet with lots of whole grains, fruits and vegetables, and yogurt.
- Yogurt with acidophilus is a great addition to the diet. Use plain yogurt and add natural sweeteners such as honey, applesauce or fruit juice.

NUTRITIONAL SUPPLEMENTS

- **Acidophilus and Bifidus:** Acidophilus contains friendly bacteria essential in fighting the fungal growth. It can be found in yogurt, liquid form or capsules.
- **Vitamin C with Bioflavonoids:** This combination helps strengthen the immune system and in healing the tissue infected with the fungus.
- **B-Complex Vitamins:** Use yeast free B-complex vitamins to help relax the nervous system, boost immunity and aid in healing damaged tissue.

- **Vitamin A/Beta-Carotene:** These help heal the tissues and stimulate function of the immune system.
- **Zinc:** Zinc helps with building immunity and in inhibiting the growth of the fungus.
- **Selenium:** This is an immune builder to help fight the fungus.
- **Chlorophyll:** Chlorophyll is full of nutrients to clean the blood and remove toxins from the body.

HERBAL REMEDIES

- **Tea Tree Oil:** Tea tree oil has been researched and found to contain anti-fungal properties. It is effective in treating skin conditions such as athlete's foot. It aids in healing and relieving the itching. It should be used mixed with warm water. (10 drops of tea tree oil to 1 quart of warm water)
- **Garlic:** Garlic can help in killing fungus. It can be taken internally in capsule form or applied directly to the rash in an extract form.
- **Black Walnut:** It may be taken internally in capsule form or used as an extract externally. It is a powerful aid in killing fungal infections.
- **Chaparral:** Chaparral is a natural antiseptic applied externally. It may also be taken internally to promote healing.
- **Myrrh:** Myrrh is an antifungal herb which can be used with warm water to wash the feet.
- **Aloe Vera:** Aloe vera gel can be applied to the area affected to soothe and heal.

ATTENTION DEFICIT DISORDER
(See Hyperactivity)

BAD BREATH

Bad breath can be a problem, causing embarrassment for children. Other children may make fun and tease a child with breath odor. It's important to correct the problem as soon as possible.

CAUSES

In some instances, bad breath may be a sign of the onset of an illness. Breath odor may also be related to certain diseases such as herpes infection, tonsillitis, diabetes, tooth decay, sinus drainage, sinus infection or strep infection. Fats that are stored in the body tissue may pass byproducts into the bloodstream and circulate to the lungs releasing gases that cause bad breath. Most often it is related to poor dental hygiene, constipation or poor digestion.

HOME CARE

- Brushing the teeth and flossing can be a first step in identifying the problem.
- Use herbs, other supplements or fiber to help relieve constipation if this is a problem.
- A stool analysis by a competent medical professional can diagnose the presence of parasites or problems with digestion and assimilation.
- Use natural breath freshening supplements.

DIETARY GUIDELINES

- Avoid sugar, refined foods and sticky fruit treats that can lead to tooth decay.

- Encourage a diet high in fiber, fruits, vegetables and whole grains.
- Chewing parsley can help freshen the breath.
- Fresh, raw fruits and vegetables can help keep the mouth fresh between brushing.

NUTRITIONAL SUPPLEMENTS

- **Chlorophyll/Blue-Green Algae:** Tablets or liquid can help freshen the breath and correct digestion problems.
- **Digestive Enzymes:** These can help with improved digestion and assimilation.
- **Acidophilus and Bifidus:** These can help keep the lower bowels functioning, improve digestion, promote friendly bacteria and reduce gas.
- **Zinc:** Some forms of bad breath may be lined to a zinc deficiency.
- **Multi-Vitamin/Mineral:** A multi-mineral and vitamin supplement can help the body eliminate toxins and function properly.

HERBAL REMEDIES

- **Aloe Vera:** Aloe Vera can help clean the digestive tract and aid in healing mouth sores.
- **Peppermint:** Tea, fresh herb or capsules can help with digestion and in freshening the breath.
- **Cascara Sagrada:** This is a natural laxative to help when constipation is a problem.
- **Bowel cleansing herbal combinations** can be used.

BEDWETTING

Bedwetting is an irritating condition which can be frustrating for both parent and child. The medical term for bedwetting is enuresis. It can be very embarrassing for the child involved. For this reason it is important for the parent not to make a big issue of the problem or get angry at the child when the bedwetting occurs. It is not a bad behavior, and the child does not even realize it is happening. The child usually has an immature or small bladder which cannot hold the fluid throughout the night.

Every child's growth and development are different. Most children outgrow the condition by the age of four or five. Boys tend to be bedwetters more than girls. Rarely does the condition persist into puberty.

CAUSES

Bedwetting can stem from either physical or psychological problems. Physically, a child may have a condition such as an inflammation of the urinary tract or some other type of disorder. This is generally a very small percentage of cases. Immature development of the nerves involved with bladder control may contribute. Psychological problems may be a factor. But this does not seem to be a common reason for bedwetting in studies done. A child who has been dry for a period of time and then starts wetting, may be suffering from a frightening event, stress or even excess fatigue.

Childhood allergies have been linked to bedwetting. Some believe the major allergens contributing to this problem are milk and milk products, wheat, eggs, corn, chocolate, and pork. Inhalants such as pollens, house dust, molds, and animal hair may also cause bedwetting. The problem seems to be associated with decreased bladder capacity due to allergies, causing inflammation and swelling. Fluid builds up layers of the bladder and cause it to swell. When the allergen is removed, the bladder will most likely return to normal size.

HOME CARE

- Use a plastic sheet under the regular sheet to make clean up easier.
- Do not make a big deal about it as the child feels bad enough.
- Try to avoid liquids after dinner or for two hours before bedtime. This may not be possible, but only allow small drinks.
- Wake the child up a few hours after bedtime to go to the bathroom.
- Be positive with the child. Encouragement is what they need.
- Do not scold or punish a child when they wet the bed.

DIETARY GUIDELINES

- Any known allergens should be removed.
- Cranberry and cherry juice can help strengthen the urinary tract. Try to find juices made with natural sweeteners rather than refined sugar. Cranberry supplements are also available.
- Try to avoid giving the child a lot to drink before bedtime.
- Avoid sugar treats or milk products before bed.
- Feed the child a nutritious diet in order to strengthen the immune system and health. Whole grains, brown rice, millet, natural foods, fruits and vegetables are beneficial.
- Fresh carrot and celery juice can help strengthen the kidneys.
- Avoid foods irritating to the kidneys such as milk, ice cream, sugar drinks, soda, caffeine drinks and chocolate.

NUTRITIONAL SUPPLEMENTS

- **Protein Drinks:** Protein drinks found in health food stores may aid in strengthening the bladder.
- **Multi-Mineral/Vitamin:** A multi-mineral/vitamin supplement can help provide essential nutrients and relieve stress.
- **Vitamins A and E:** These help to normalize bladder muscle function.
- **Potassium:** A supplement can help with fluid balance and kidney function.
- **Calcium/Magnesium:** This combination can help the child relax and reduce stress which may be a contributing factor.
- **Silicon/Zinc:** These can help in strengthening the bladder.

HERBAL REMEDIES

- **Uva Ursi:** This is strengthening and healing to the urinary tract.
- **Buchu:** Buchu can also help build the urinary tract.
- **Parsley:** Parsley is a natural diuretic which can improve bladder muscle tone.
- **Plantain:** Plantain helps strengthen the kidneys and bladder.
- **Herbal combinations** can also be helpful and some contain Juniper Berries, Golden Seal, Watermelon Seed, etc.
- **Herbal combinations** for the nervous system may help children who are nervous and sensitive.

BEHAVIORAL PROBLEMS

Behavioral problems occur in children for various reasons. But one thing that most parents of children with behavioral disorders have in common is that they often feel despair. It often appears that some children with behavioral disorders want to make others lives miserable around them. They may look for opportunities to disrupt a situation. These children need to find peace within themselves and learn to deal with their personal difficulties. There are natural methods which can help along with parents, siblings, teachers, counselors and others. Some types of behavioral disorders are as follows:

Aggression, which is a natural part of a personality, can become out of control and turn into violent behavior. Some children want to hurt themselves and others as well. Violent outbursts may occur without provocation when a child is at play. One small problem may set them off. They may not have the ability to control the feelings of anger which can turn into a violent rage.

Tantrums occur in all children from time to time. But frequent attacks may be the sign of a problem. Loud screaming and yelling are usually part of a tantrum. They may occur when a child is trying to get attention.

Breath holding can be a frightening experience for any parent. A child may do it the first time in a rage. Then seeing the reaction of the parent, may continue the behavior for attention. The child may lose consciousness for a few moments and then awake breathing normally.

Hyperactivity can occur in children for various reasons. Some children become so wound up there seems to be no way of controlling them. These type of children are hard to be around for prolonged periods because they tend to annoy everyone within range.

CAUSES

Stomach and digestion problems can make a child feel uncomfortable and sometimes this discomfort can be reflected in negative behavior. Toxins may cause similar discomfort and behavior. Allergies are another common concern. Check to see if the child is allergic to certain foods or substances. This can be a cause of negative behavior because the child feels awful. Children who do not feel well may not be able to identify the cause. It is important to examine the behavior, look for possible causes and seek professional help if necessary. Negative behavior should be stopped as soon as possible to avoid escalation of the problem.

Behavioral problems may stem from emotional causes. Stress and tension at home are sensed by the child. They do not have the emotional maturity to recognize or identify what is bothering them. Children that are close to their parents will often reflect the emotions of the parent.

HOME CARE

- Encourage the child to take responsibility for their behavior.
- Reward good behavior, and avoid, as much as possible, negative behavior.
- Encourage healthy, regular eating habits. Low blood sugar problems may be a factor.
- Exercise is helpful for burning excess energy. Go for a walk, hike, bike ride, or play in the backyard or park. It is also a good way to focus energy positively and learn appropriate behavior.
- Do not give up. Patience and consistency are essential when trying to correct negative behavior.

DIETARY GUIDELINES

- Diet is often a factor in behavior disorders.
- Make sure regular meals are served. Low blood sugar can cause mood swings.
- Avoid common foods which are related to allergies such as milk and milk products, nuts, sugar, artificial colorings and flavorings, preservatives, and wheat products.
- Serve whole, natural foods, vegetables, fruit, and lots of pure water.

NUTRITIONAL SUPPLEMENTS

- **B-Complex:** The B-complex vitamins are soothing to the nervous system. They are essential for brain function.
- **Calcium/Magnesium:** This combination is necessary for proper nerve function and for a healthy body. They have a calming effect on the body.
- **Vitamin C:** Vitamin C is essential to a healthy body and for healing. It is important in the synthesis of neurotransmitters in the brain.
- **Essential Fatty Acids:** EFA's are important in a child's diet. They are found in the membranes around each cell. They are important for all body functions and the immune system.

HERBAL REMEDIES

- **Chamomile:** Chamomile is calming and relaxing to the nervous system.
- **Ginkgo:** Ginkgo is important for the function of the brain.

- **Gotu Kola:** This is considered a brain food and may help with mental function.
- **Passion Flower:** Passion Flower is relaxing and can help with insomnia.

BITES AND STINGS

There is no way to avoid a child getting bit by a mosquito or stung by a bee. Any child who likes to be outdoors is vulnerable. Whether you live in the city or the country or anywhere in between, bugs abound. The most common culprits include mosquitoes, bees, gnats, fleas, spiders, and ants. They cause swelling, itching and sometimes pain. Usually, these are only an annoyance, but some are more serious. A severe allergic reaction to a bee sting should be dealt with immediately. Black widow or brown recluse spider bites should receive emergency treatment. Deer tick bites can lead to serious conditions such as Lyme disease and Rocky Mountain Spotted Fever.

CAUSES

The cause involves being bitten or stung by an insect of some type. It is impossible to fully avoid exposure to insects and so treatment should be given as needed. The area should be cleaned with soap and water. An icepack or cold compress can help relieve swelling. Medical treatment should be sought if pain is severe. Bee stings should be removed with tweezers. An antiseptic should be applied to both stings and bites. A paste of baking soda and water can help soothe the area.

Home Care

- Apply a baking soda paste to the affected area.
- Watch for signs of infection such as inflammation, tenderness and redness.
- A cold compress can be soothing and reduce the inflammation.
- If stung by a bee, check to make sure the stinger is gone.
- If the child shows any sign of distress, such as shock, extreme pain or listlessness, or if a poisonous insect bite is suspected, get medical attention immediately.
- Bee and wasp stings can be treated with crushed charcoal tablets applied with a cotton ball.
- Light colored, plain clothing is less attractive to insects.

Dietary Guidelines

- Plenty of fluids should be given to help flush out any residual toxins. Pure water, juices, and soups can be given.
- Individuals who eat high sugar diets seem to be more attractive to insects.

Nutritional Supplements

- **Calcium:** Calcium, either in liquid or tablet form, may help ease the pain.
- **Vitamin B1:** Studies have shown that individuals who have diets high in vitamin B1 or take a supplement are less attractive to insects.
- **Vitamin C:** Vitamin C is healing to insect bite and sting wounds.
- **Clay Pack:** A clay paste can be applied to the affected area to help draw out the poisons and soothe itching and pain.

HERBAL REMEDIES

- **Aloe Vera:** Aloe Vera is soothing and healing to skin irritations.
- **Echinacea:** Echinacea is healing and can help prevent infection.
- **Comfrey:** A poultice can help draw out the poisons, reduce swelling and promote healing.
- **Chickweed:** A cream (ointment) with chickweed can help soothe and heal.
- **Garlic and Onion:** Eating garlic and onion may help repel insects. They don't seem to like the odor. Of course, your friends might not either.
- **Witch Hazel:** Witch Hazel can be applied to the area to relieve inflammation and itching.
- **Lobelia:** Lobelia extract can be applied to the area to clean, soothe and draw out the poisons.
- **Tea Tree Oil:** This is healing and soothing.
- **Black Walnut:** Black Walnut works as an antiseptic and to draw out toxins.

BLEEDING

Children will experience an injury involving bleeding sometime during their early years. The severity will vary due to the seriousness of the injury. Always be calm to reassure the child that everything will be fine.

For minor scrapes and cuts, wash the area with soap and water. Apply pressure if necessary to stop the bleeding. Tea tree oil will help disinfect the area. Cover with a bandage.

More serious injuries require extra care. Apply pressure with a sterile cloth, if possible, immediately, and elevate the area that is bleeding. Apply more dressings if the area continues to bleed. Seek medical attention for serious injuries, as stitches may be necessary.

CAUSES

The causes vary from a fall on the sidewalk to a major accident. Each should be treated appropriately. Some children seem to be more accident prone than others. Active children generally receive more scrapes and cuts. Excessive bleeding may be due to nutrient deficiencies such as calcium and vitamin K.

HOME CARE

- If bleeding is severe, seek medical attention immediately.
- Keep the affected area clean to avoid infection.
- Watch for signs of infection.

DIETARY GUIDELINES

- When blood loss occurs, green leafy vegetables, other vegetables and fresh fruits are helpful in providing vitamins and minerals essential to health and healing.
- A natural food diet can help in healing.
- Citrus juices can help strengthen the capillaries.

NUTRITIONAL SUPPLEMENTS

- **Iron:** may be recommended for serious blood loss. Constipation may occur; if so, add fiber to the diet.
- **Vitamin C with Bioflavonoids:** This is useful for healing and strengthening the capillaries. They help to reduce inflammation and aid the immune system.
- **Chlorophyll:** Chlorophyll is full of nutrients for health and can help build the blood after a loss.
- **B-Complex Vitamins:** This combination can help in the healing process.
- **Vitamin A:** Vitamin A is healing to the body tissues.

HERBAL REMEDIES

- **Aloe Vera:** This can help soothe and heal minor injuries.
- **Burdock:** Burdock is high in natural iron.
- **Yellow Dock:** Yellow Dock helps in building healthy blood.
- **Capsicum:** This can help stop bleeding. A combination of one teaspoon capsicum in one cup of hot water can help stop nosebleeds.

BOILS

A boil is an infection that begins beneath the surface of the skin in the hair follicles. They are painful, irritating and can leave scars. The bacteria most commonly causing boils is *Staphylococcus aureus*. Boils can be found most often on the neck, face, under the arms or buttocks. They can be found singly or in groups. Boils usually begin as a red, raised bump that may become painful and form a pustule within a few days. The infection may, in rare cases, spread to the lymph system and require medical attention.

CAUSES

Boils happen when the bacteria invades a hair follicle or a break in the skin. Inflammation and pus develop as the infection is fought by the body. Boils can be a sign of a weak immune system. They sometimes occur in individuals who have diabetes or when there is poor hygiene. Skin disorders may also be found when constipation is a problem and toxins enter the bloodstream. Other factors which may increase the risk of boils are stress, allergies, poor diet, certain drugs, infection, and thyroid problems.

HOME CARE

- Do not attempt to squeeze or incise a boil. This should be done by a qualified medical professional.
- Warm compresses can be applied to the boil until it comes to a head and ruptures on its own. A warm clay pack can also be applied to help draw toxins out of the area.
- If the boil is accompanied by a fever, irritability, loss of appetite or listlessness, seek medical attention.

- Wash hands thoroughly after touching the area to avoid spreading the condition.
- Soak the boil in Epsom salt to help bring the abscess to a head.
- Wash the area several times a day and apply an antiseptic.
- Honey can help when applied directly to the boil, according to an article in *Lancet*, January 9, 1993.

DIETARY GUIDELINES

- Avoid refined sugars and fats as they can lower the immune response and leave the body susceptible to infection.
- Fruits and vegetables, especially dark green leafy vegetables, are full of nutritional value for healing.
- Fresh carrot and celery juice can help healing.

NUTRITIONAL SUPPLEMENTS

- **Vitamin A/Beta-Carotene:** These will help improve immune function and aid in healing. A vitamin A capsule can be opened and applied directly to the area.
- **Vitamin C and Bioflavonoids:** These help healing, reduce inflammation, and boost the immune system.
- **Chlorophyll/Blue-Green Algae:** These offer nutritional support and rid the bloodstream of toxins.
- **Vitamin E:** This can help with healing, to strengthen the immune system and to reduce scarring. It can be applied directly to the affected area.
- **Zinc:** A zinc supplement can help support healing and the immune system. Avoid prolonged usage and follow directions given on label.

HERBAL REMEDIES

- **Tea Tree Oil:** This can be applied directly to the area to kill the bacteria.
- **Burdock:** Burdock can help cleanse the blood and works as a natural antibiotic.
- **Aloe Vera:** Aloe vera gel can help heal and reduce scarring.
- **Ginger:** A ginger tea compress can help draw out toxins.
- **Echinacea:** This is a natural antibiotic and builds the immune function.
- **Garlic:** Garlic is a natural antibiotic to promote healing.
- **Milk Thistle, Flaxseed, Black Walnut and Slippery Elm:** These all help to draw out poisons when applied as a hot poultice to the boil.
- **Herbal blood cleanser and bowel combinations** can help.

BROKEN BONES

Broken bones require immediate medical attention. Bones are living components of the body, and a break can be extremely painful. Children's bones may heal quickly, but they require medical treatment in order to ensure proper development and growth. There may be a wound at the sight of the fracture. It will be tender and may be swollen and red. Immobilize the area if possible while seeking medical attention. Be careful with head, neck and spinal injuries, and avoid moving the child. Natural remedies can help with the discomfort and recovery process.

CAUSES

A fall or any accident can cause a fracture. Teach children to be careful and avoid dangerous situations. But this will probably not always work for many children. Active children are apt to be in situations where injuries such as broken bones are a possibility. In fact, many fractures occur in seemingly harmless situations. No one can be entirely protected from injury.

HOME CARE

- Seek medical attention.
- Do not move a child if a serious fracture is suspected such as vertebra, skull, neck or back injury. Call for emergency help.
- Reassure the child by remaining calm and talking in a soothing tone.
- Apply ice to less serious fractures involving small bones, fingers, and toes to reduce swelling and relieve pain.

DIETARY GUIDELINES

- The child should be given healthy, nutritious foods such as whole grains, fruits and vegetables and plenty of calcium rich food.
- Avoid sugar and soda which can leach calcium from the bones. Soda is high in phosphorus which can use up calcium necessary for bone support.
- Brown rice is nutritious and high in calcium and magnesium.
- Almonds are good to munch on for older children and contain fiber, calcium and magnesium. Almond milk can be given to younger children.

NUTRITIONAL SUPPLEMENTS

- **Calcium:** A calcium supplement will help heal and strengthen the structural system.
- **Magnesium:** Magnesium is needed to help with calcium absorption. It works with the body to transfer calcium from the blood into the bones.
- **Multi-Mineral Supplement:** A multi-mineral supplement is necessary for strong bones and teeth.
- **Vitamin A:** It is healing and helps in rebuilding tissue.
- **Vitamin D:** Vitamin D helps with the absorption of calcium in the body.
- **Essential Fatty Acids:** Often lacking in the diet of children are EFA's. They are essential for all functions of the body and should be supplemented.
- **Chlorophyll:** Chlorophyll is full of trace minerals necessary for rebuilding tissue.

HERBAL REMEDIES

- **Horsetail:** Horsetail has been researched and found to contain silica which helps promote healthy bone and tissue growth. A supplement would be helpful after a bone injury. It may not be recommended for young children.
- **Oatstraw:** Oatstraw is also high in silica which aids in healing and strengthening bones.
- **Comfrey:** This is an herb useful for helping strengthen the structural system. It is high in calcium and other minerals and vitamins essential for bone repair.

BRUISES

Bruising occurs when an injury causes a blood vessel to leak into the tissues surrounding the affected area. The skin is not broken, but the underlying area is injured. Discoloration occurs with the blood collecting under the skin area. The degree of bruising depends upon the severity of the injury. Recovery usually occurs without medical intervention. The tiny vessels heal quickly as the body reabsorbs the blood from the injury.

CAUSES

Bruises are the result of a fall or injury to the skin and small capillaries below the surface of the skin. This is a very common injury and no child can grow and develop without a variety of bruises. A bruise usually starts as a red, swollen area gradually changing to black, blue and yellow as healing occurs. Severe bruising from mild injuries may be a symptom of serious conditions such as anemia, malnutrition, leukemia, and blood clotting disorders.

HOME CARE

- Apply ice to the bruised area.
- Watch a child carefully if they have suffered a blow to the head area.
- Avoid using aspirin.
- Visit a health care professional if bruising occurs frequently.

DIETARY GUIDELINES

- A healthy diet should be followed containing whole grains, fruits and vegetables, allowing for nutrients to aid in the healing process.
- Dark, green leafy vegetables are full of nutrients.

NUTRITIONAL SUPPLEMENTS

- **Vitamin C with Bioflavonoids:** Vitamin C and bioflavonoids aid in healing and strengthening the body. They help in supporting the blood vessels and capillaries.
- **Vitamin A:** This vitamin is healing and can help the tissues repair.
- **B-Complex:** B-Complex vitamins can help protect the tissues.
- **Vitamin E:** Vitamin E can help heal and strengthen the veins.
- **Calcium and Magnesium:** These will help with healing.
- **Zinc:** Zinc is useful in the healing process. Follow directions for children on label.
- **Chlorophyll/Blue-Green Algae:** It is full of nutrients and minerals to promote healing and strengthen the veins.

HERBAL REMEDIES

- **Alfalfa:** Alfalfa is full of nutrients and minerals to aid in healing the body.
- **Horsetail:** Horsetail can help repair damaged tissue. It is not recommended for younger children.
- **Kelp:** Kelp contains nutrients to aid in healing.
- **White Oak Bark:** It is high in calcium which aids in healing.
- **Black Walnut, Comfrey and Aloe Vera:** A warm poultice using these herbs can help promote healing.

BURNS

Burns vary in degree as to their severity and seriousness. First degree burns will cause redness, mild swelling and pain. Second degree burns will cause redness and blistering. Third degree cause destruction of the skin and underlying muscle tissue. Little pain occurs because the nerve endings are destroyed. Small children should be supervised at all times to avoid the possibility of a burn injury.

CAUSES

Burns range from mild to charring with destruction of all layers of the skin. Any time the skin surface is in contact with heat, a burn may occur. Even the sun can cause burning. A sunburn can be serious and exposure to the sun should be gradual and sunscreen is advised. Steam, fire and chemical burns can all cause serious damage. Children should be supervised at all times around hot surfaces. A small child can accidentally turn on the hot water if left alone or pull a hot pan from the stove, causing serious injury.

First degree burns usually result from the sun or hot water.

Second degree burns usually occur from hot metal objects, flame contact or severe sunburns.

Third degree burns are the result of high flame contact, hot fluid burns, steam from a pressure cooker, X-rays, and electrical burns which can cause death.

Fourth degree burns can cause total destruction of the skin and can also destroy organic bodily functions and may be fatal.

Cold water should be applied until the pain has subsided. Cold water can help stop the burning process and may prevent blistering. Clothes that cover the burn should not be removed but soaked to prevent further burning. Blisters should not be broken because they offer protection from infection to the delicate skin tissue.

HOME CARE

- Apply cold water to the area.
- Elevate the area to reduce swelling and pain.
- Do not break blisters as it may lead to infection.
- Keep the affected area dry and clean, usually covered with gauze.
- Cucumber juice applied to sunburns and other burns can help with soothing and healing.

DIETARY GUIDELINES

- Pure water is helpful in providing fluids to the body tissue.
- Fruits and vegetables are cleansers and contain nutrients essential to healing.
- Green drinks are healing.

NUTRITIONAL SUPPLEMENTS

- **Vitamin A and Beta-Carotene:** These will both help speed the healing process.
- **B-Complex:** The B-complex vitamins are helpful in healing.
- **Vitamin C with Bioflavonoids:** This will help with healing, inflammation, strengthening the immune system and preventing infection.
- **Potassium:** Potassium will help maintain fluid and electrolyte balance.
- **Vitamin E:** It is healing used externally and internally.
- **Multi-Mineral Supplement:** Minerals will help with healing and repairing tissue.

- **Honey:** Honey is healing, and when applied to the area, can reduce the risk of infection.

Herbal Remedies

- **Comfrey:** Comfrey helps with new cell growth. A salve can be applied to the injury. A poultice of comfrey, wheat germ oil and honey can be applied to the burn to promote healing and new skin growth. A gauze can be lightly applied to the burn.
- **Slippery Elm:** This is healing, builds new cells and draws toxins from the body.
- **Golden Seal:** Golden seal will help in preventing infection and healing.
- **Aloe Vera:** Aloe vera is healing and soothing on burns.
- **Horsetail:** Horsetail is healing and promotes tissue growth.

CANCER

Cancer is a frightening thought for parents with children. It often brings painful memories and fear. But the fact remains that cancer is the number one killer of children. More babies and children are developing cancer than ever before. It is estimated that one in three individuals will develop cancer at sometime during their life. The American Cancer Society has reported that cancer is the leading cause of death in children under the age of fifteen in the United States. Leukemia and lymphoma were the major cancers attributing to fifty percent of the deaths. Cancer of the brain and central nervous system, soft tissues, kidney and bone accounted for the remaining deaths.

CAUSES

A poor diet in a pregnant mother, along with negative life style habits may increase the vulnerability in infants of developing cancer. Smoking by the mother can cause a lower immune system function in infants and children. The fetus is vulnerable to toxins, chemicals, air pollution, drugs and even aspirin. Certain chemicals such as benzopyrene, arsenic and chemicals found in smog can cause immune impairment in the fetus and children. Asbestos can lead to a cancer known as mesothelioma. This cancer involves the pleurae, the covering of the lungs and the peritoneum and the covering of the abdominal organs. Asbestos fibers are found in older schools, homes and office buildings. They are known to cause cancer and other problems. Inherited weaknesses can cause cellular degeneration. But with a healthy life style, cancer risk can be lessened. Diets low in fiber and high in proteins, and fats, as well as mineral imbalance, and a lack of vitamins can cause cancer cells to grow. Autointoxication from chronic constipation and fermentation in the intestines may also contribute to cancer. Stress can weaken the body, and along with a poor diet, can predispose an individual to cancer.

HOME CARE

- Pregnant women need to be sure and eat a healthy diet for themselves and their baby.
- Avoid x-rays during pregnancy.
- A positive attitude can help. Cancer does not have to be fatal.
- Be calm around the child. Do not let them feel your fear.
- Protect children as much as possible from emotional upsets.
- Avoid constipation in children.

DIETARY GUIDELINES

- Avoid dairy products. They can cause excess mucus which is a breeding ground for germs and viruses.
- Avoid junk foods, refined foods, saturated fats, sugar, and white flour.
- Limit meat intake and fats. Some fats, when heated, contain cancer causing properties.
- Feed children ample amounts of vegetables such as carrots, spinach, and sweet potatoes. They contain beta-carotene which has shown to reduce the risk of cancer of the lungs, larynx, esophagus, stomach, colon, rectum, prostate and urinary system.
- Cruciferous vegetables have been linked to lower risk of cancer. These include broccoli, Brussel's sprouts, cabbage, cauliflower, kohlrabi and kale.
- Feed children foods high in fiber such as grains, millet, oatmeal, beans, nuts and seeds. A high fiber diet has been linked to a lower incidence of cancer.
- Nitrates and nitrites are suspected in some cases of leukemia. They are found in hot dogs, lunch meat and many processed foods.
- Drink juices such as beet, carrot, asparagus, cabbage, grape, black cherry and fresh apple.
- Eat onions and garlic.
- Almonds are high in laetrile which has been known to have anti-cancer properties.

NUTRITIONAL SUPPLEMENTS

- **Vitamin A and Beta-Carotene:** These help fight free radicals found in the food we eat, the air we breathe, and rancid foods.
- **Vitamin C and Bioflavonoids:** These help protect against cancer and protect the immune system. They are needed on a daily basis.

- **Vitamin E:** This is an antioxidant vitamin to protect against free radical damage and immune related diseases such as cancer.
- **B-Complex Vitamins:** The B vitamins help protect the liver, aid in digestion, help strengthen the nervous system and eliminate toxins.
- **Essential Fatty Acids:** The essential fatty acids help protect against cancer and strengthen the immune system. Many children may be lacking in these.
- **Selenium and Zinc:** These are important as antioxidants. They help strengthen the immune system and protect against cancer.
- **Chlorophyll/Blue-Green Algae:** These contain important cancer fighting nutrients.
- **Indoles:** Dietary indoles can be found in children's combinations. They help to strengthen the immune system to prevent diseases such as cancer.

HERBAL REMEDIES

- **Burdock:** Burdock is a blood cleanser and contains properties that can prevent tumor growth.
- **Echinacea:** This improves the function of the immune system. It helps the body produce interferon to protect against cancer and purifies the blood and lymphatic system.
- **Fenugreek:** Fenugreek helps to clean mucus and toxins from the body.
- **Garlic:** Garlic is a natural antibiotic and protects and strengthens the immune system.
- **Kelp:** Kelp is rich in minerals to protect the immune system.
- **Pau D'Arco:** Pau D'Arco helps clean the blood and protects against cancers of all kinds.
- **Red Clover:** Red Clover is an excellent blood cleanser and protects against cancer.

115

- **Rose Hips:** Rose Hips are rich in vitamin C which helps protect the immune system.
- **Suma:** Suma helps protect against cancer.
- **Yellow Dock:** Yellow Dock is rich in iron and helps purify the blood and liver.

CHICKENPOX

Chickenpox is a common childhood illness. It usually begins with a slight fever and headache. It is characterized by skin eruptions beginning as small red spots and, over a period of a few hours, blistering and breaking, eventually scabbing. The incubation period is between two to three weeks. The older the child, the worse case they may receive of chickenpox. It usually occurs in children between the ages of five and nine. A few adults will get chickenpox if they avoided the illness as a child.

CAUSES

Chickenpox is a virus known as Varicella-zoster. It spreads from person to person, usually children, through airborne droplets or through direct contact. Chickenpox are highly contagious during the two day period before the rash develops and for about a week after until all the spots have scabbed. Spots will probably continue to develop for a few days. Full recovery takes about two weeks. When the scabs are gone, the child is no longer contagious. The rash will itch, but the child should be encouraged not to scratch because scars may develop and infection can occur. Healthy children will get chickenpox. It is a way to rid toxins from the body that build up through toxins from foods and the environment. Rare complications may occur such as infection, encephalitis

116

and pneumonia. Aspirin should not be given to children because of the risk of Reye's syndrome.

HOME CARE

- Keep the child's nails trimmed to avoid scratching.
- The child can soak in a bath with 1 cup baking soda, and 1/2 cup apple cider vinegar. This can help with the itching.
- A bath with chamomile will also help itching.
- Vitamin E can be applied to the scar after the scab has fallen off.
- A warm bath can help the rash to appear sooner. Burdock and Golden Seal can be added to the bath water.

DIETARY GUIDELINES

- Avoid sugar, processed foods, additives and fatty foods to help build the immune system.
- Offer plenty of pure water, fruit and vegetable juices.
- Mild foods may be preferred if sores occur in the mouth.
- Fruit juice popsicles and nutritious shakes may be appealing to the child.
- Avoid spicy foods.
- Fresh fruit and vegetable juices can be given.
- Lemon or lime juice sweetened with honey will help cleanse the blood.
- Potato broth and onion soup will provide nutrients for healing.

NUTRITIONAL SUPPLEMENTS

- **Vitamin A and Beta-Carotene:** These will help enhance the immune system and heal tissue.
- **Vitamin C:** Vitamin C will help with healing, in reducing fever, and to help with viral infections.
- **Vitamin E:** This is useful in healing and building the immune system.
- **Multi-Mineral Supplement:** Essential minerals help with healing and electrolyte balance.
- **Chlorophyll/Blue-Green Algae:** Chlorophyll can help purify the blood of toxins.

HERBAL REMEDIES

- **Aloe Vera:** Aloe Vera can be applied externally to the sores to promote healing and soothe the itching.
- **Catnip:** Catnip can help calm the nerves and relax the child.
- **Ginger:** Ginger is useful for childhood complaints such as chickenpox.
- **Chamomile:** Chamomile will help induce sleep and relaxation.
- **Comfrey:** A salve with comfrey can help relieve itching and soothe the area.
- **Golden Seal:** It will help prevent infection, promote healing, and prevent itching.
- **Red Clover:** Red Clover is a blood purifier.
- **Yarrow:** This will help with the healing process.
- **Cascara Sagrada:** Cascara Sagrada or other herbal laxatives can be given to aid in cleaning toxins from the body.

COLD SORES / CANKER SORES

Cold sores are similar to canker sores but cold sores are usually around the dry lip area and canker sores are commonly seen inside the mouth and lip. They both are very painful and a cure has never been found. Shortening the duration of the eruption may be possible. They are painful and irritating and may last up to two weeks. They usually heal on their own, and there is very little that can be done once an eruption occurs.

CAUSES

The cause of canker and cold sores is not entirely known. They are both viral in nature and may be passed from mother to child during the first few months of birth. Heredity also seems to play a role because they tend to run in families. Cold sores are known as herpes simplex type 1. Both of these conditions usually are dormant in the body until there is a stressful situation causing the immune system to be lowered. This may occur when there is a cold, during menstruation, exposure to certain foods, or under stress.

HOME CARE

- Sucking on ice may help relieve some of the pain associated with cold and canker sores. Apply ice to cold sores for about thirty minutes at the first sign of eruption.
- Hydrogen peroxide can be applied to the area using a cotton swab.
- A wet tea bag may be applied to the area to relieve pain.
- Rinse the mouth with baking soda. It can help reduce acidity.

Dietary Guidelines

- Avoid foods that may cause allergic reactions such as walnuts, citrus fruits, and chocolate.
- A diet high in fresh, leafy green vegetables and onions may be beneficial.
- Yogurt with acidophilus can help heal and prevent eruptions.
- Foods high in vitamin C such as cranberry juice, broccoli, and cantaloupe are helpful.
- A raw potato, which contains vitamin P, placed directly on the sore may promote the healing process.
- Cabbage juice may help in healing.
- Avoid acidic foods when an eruption is present.

Nutritional Supplements

- **Antioxidant Vitamins:** The antioxidant nutrients (C, Beta-Carotene, E) are important for strengthening the immune system. As these conditions may be related to immune function, promoting immune function may be beneficial.
- **B-Complex Vitamins:** The B-complex vitamins are essential to the nervous system. They are also helpful in healing and promoting immune function. A lack of the B vitamins has been linked to outbreaks.
- **Vitamin C:** Vitamin C is important in boosting the immune system, healing and repairing tissue damage.
- **Vitamin E:** Vitamin E is healing and can be applied to the sore directly.
- **Vitamin A and Beta-Carotene:** These can be taken to speed the healing process.
- **Acidophilus and Bifidus:** Acidophilus can help replenish the friendly bacteria in the body to improve healing.

- **L-Lysine:** L-Lysine deficiencies can be a factor in the outbreak of the sores.
- **Indoles:** Dietary indoles, often found in children's combinations, can help strengthen the immune system.

HERBAL REMEDIES

- **Golden Seal:** Golden Seal may be used as a mouthwash or applied directly to the sore. It can help prevent infection and heal the area.
- **Aloe Vera:** Aloe Vera may be applied directly to the sore to aid in the healing process.
- **Echinacea:** Echinacea is strengthening to the immune system and aids in healing and preventing infection.
- **Licorice:** Licorice root tea can be used as a mouthwash. It has antiviral and antibacterial properties to promote healing.
- **Myrrh:** Drops of Myrrh can be added to water and applied to the area to promote healing.
- **Lobelia:** Lobelia extract can be applied to the sore area to promote healing and reduce pain.

COLIC

Colic is a common condition in babies. It may be related to their immature digestive systems, causing gas and pain in the abdominal area. It seems to be cramping of the abdomen from indigestion or gas pains. It is usually associated with lengthy periods of crying when the baby cannot be consoled. What differentiates colic from other problems is the sudden onset of prolonged crying with arched back and tense body. It is most common during the first four months of life but may continue longer in some infants.

CAUSES

Bottle fed babies are more prone to colic. Sucking in air with formula may contribute to the gas pains. Allergies to milk protein either in the formula or from breast feeding due to food the mother is ingesting may cause colic. Tension on the part of the mother or father may result in a tense baby. Try and relax, especially during feeding time. Not adequately burping a baby after feeding may result in bouts of colic. Overfeeding an infant may cause stomach cramping. Poor elimination may cause stomach cramping and pain. Medical professionals do not know what causes colic or why some babies suffer from the condition and others seem immune.

HOME CARE

- Take the baby for a ride in the car to relax and induce sleep. Leave him in his car seat when you get home, if necessary, to avoid waking the child.
- Burp the baby every few minutes during feeding.
- Relax when holding the child. They sense tension in caregivers.
- Place a warm bottle between your lap and the baby's abdomen.
- Rock or walk the infant.
- Baby swings may help comfort and relax the baby.
- Be careful not to overfeed the child.
- Make sure the baby's feet are kept warm as cold feet are thought to cause abdominal pain.
- Massage the baby's abdomen clockwise to help relieve pain.
- Warm molasses water can help.
- A chiropractor may help if the spine is out of adjustment due to the birth process.

DIETARY GUIDELINES

- If breastfeeding, avoid dairy products and other foods which may cause problems such as chocolate, caffeine, broccoli, cauliflower, peppers, beans and spicy foods.
- If bottle feeding, check the formula the baby is taking. Maybe a change in formula will help the problem. Check with the baby's physician.
- Try using a bottle that allows less air to be sucked by the baby. Sit and hold the baby during feedings.

NUTRITIONAL SUPPLEMENTS

- **Acidophilus and Bifidus:** These may help in digestion. If breastfeeding, the mother can take the acidophilus supplement. Babies can take a small amount in the formula. (1/8 teaspoon in 8 ounce bottle of milk twice a day)

HERBAL REMEDIES

- **Chamomile:** A teaspoon of tea can be given to a colicky baby. A nursing mother can drink a cup of tea.
- **Peppermint:** Peppermint tea aids in the digestion process. A teaspoon can be given to the baby a few times a day, and nursing mothers can drink the tea.
- **Catnip:** Catnip tea is often used to help release gas, soothe and relax the muscles.
- **Red Raspberry, Spearmint, Chamomile, Orange Peel and Blue Vervain combination** in extract form may help when diluted and given in small amounts.

COMMON COLD

Billions of dollars are spent each year on trying to suppress the symptoms associated with the common cold. Children develop colds more often than adults because their immune systems are not fully developed. A cold involves the upper respiratory tract and may be associated with runny eyes, runny nose, headache, congestion, sore throat, fever, sneezing and wheezing. The average child gets approximately five colds a year. Younger children usually are more susceptible. Colds usually are less of a problem with age as immunity increases. The frequency of colds probably increases during the winter months because of the confinement and close exposure to others with the virus. There is no cure for the common cold, and antibiotics are not effective against viruses. A cold generally lasts about a week. If it lasts longer, it may be the flu, which usually causes more discomfort than a cold. The common cold is difficult to cure because of the ability of the virus to change in size and shape and can take many different forms.

CAUSES

The common cold is viral in nature and almost impossible to cure because of its ability to change into different forms. It involves the upper respiratory tract. The virus is passed from individual to individual through contact with hands, sneezing, or coughing. Children are not even aware that they are passing their illness. Poor eating habits, stress, and toxins can lower the body's resistance. A cold may be nature's way of cleaning the body by eliminating toxins. A cold generally occurs when the immune system is lowered. So improving the diet, herbal remedies and supplements may help prevent colds from developing by increasing the immune response. It may be important for a cold to run its course through all five stages of inflammation which include incubation, aggravation, destruction, absorption and reconstruction according to Louise Tenney in her book *Nutritional Guide With Food Combining,* on page 7.

HOME CARE

- Begin treating the illness at the first sign of a cold.
- Encourage rest to help conserve energy for healing.
- If the child wants to play, make sure he stays warm.
- Use a cool mist humidifier in the child's room.

DIETARY GUIDELINES

- When the child is ill, offer diluted juices, herbal teas, soups and applesauce.
- Avoid sugar and processed foods. Sugar depletes essential nutrients from the body needed for immune function.
- Warm fluids can help alleviate congestion.
- Constipation may be a problem, so encourage fiber foods.
- Citrus fruits can help clean the blood and stimulate liver function.

NUTRITIONAL SUPPLEMENTS

- **Vitamin A and Beta-Carotene:** These will help stimulate immune function, promote healing and protect the mucous membranes in the body.
- **Vitamin C and Bioflavonoids:** Some studies indicate that these will help shorten the duration of the cold as well as destroy the virus. They are healing and contain antiviral properties.

- **Zinc:** Zinc lozenges can be given to boost the immune system at the first sign of a cold. It may help reduce cold symptoms and promote healing.
- **Selenium:** Selenium may speed the healing process.
- **Chlorophyll:** This will help clear toxins from the body.

Herbal Remedies

- **Catnip:** Catnip tea can be given to children to reduce fevers and loosen congestion.
- **Chamomile:** Chamomile tea will help the child relax and rest.
- **Comfrey and Fenugreek:** This combination can help relieve congestion and control a cough.
- **Echinacea:** Echinacea is healing and stimulates immune function. It is also a natural antibiotic effective in fighting viral infections.
- **Garlic:** Garlic contains antibacterial properties and can help in healing.
- **Ginger:** Ginger can help increase perspiration and reduce fevers.
- **Golden Seal:** Golden Seal is a natural antibiotic and helps in healing.
- **Hops:** Hops can help relax and promote sleep.
- **Astragalus:** Astragalus is a Chinese herb used to reduce the length and prevent colds from occurring.
- **Cascara Sagrada:** Cascara Sagrada and other herbal laxatives can help remove toxins through the intestinal system.
- **Herbal combinations** for infection and expectorants can help with a cold.

CONJUNCTIVITIS / PINK EYE

Conjunctivitis is an inflammation of the conjunctiva which are the thin layers of tissue covering the eye and the eyelid. It is a viral infection which may turn into a secondary bacterial infection. Crusting of the eyes may occur during sleep. This can be frightening to a child, and the eye should be bathed with water and wiped gently with a clean cloth to remove the discharge. The eyes will appear red and swollen. The child will complain of burning and itching and may rub the eyes continually. The condition usually lasts about a week.

CAUSES

Conjunctivitis is a contagious-usually viral-disease often spread from family member to family member or around a classroom. It may begin with a child wiping his nose with a hand and then rubbing his eyes. It may also start a an eye irritation involving allergic reactions to things such as smoke, pollution, or something in the eye. A newborn can suffer from clogged tear ducts which in some cases is a reaction to silver nitrate put in the eyes of newborns. The clogged tear ducts allow fluid to accumulate inside the eye and often become infected. The child usually outgrows the condition in a few months. Massage the area around the tear duct a few times a day. But if the condition persists, surgery may be done to open the tear ducts.

When conjunctivitis is suspected, avoid sharing towels or pillowcases with the individual infected. Wash these after each use. The eye can be washed with a solution of 1/2 teaspoon salt to 1 cup of warm water as often as desired.

HOME CARE

- Apply a compress, using eyebright, to the eye area.
- Wash clothing, pillowcases and towels daily.
- Make sure the child washes his hands often to avoid infecting others and reinfecting himself.
- Encourage the child to avoid touching the eyes.

DIETARY GUIDELINES

- Avoid sugar and refined products. The body becomes more acidic and susceptible to infection.
- Encourage foods high in fiber and immune building vitamins and minerals.
- Green leafy vegetables, green and yellow vegetables, fruits and whole grains are beneficial.
- Pure water and juices can help in flushing toxins from the body.

NUTRITIONAL SUPPLEMENTS

- **Vitamin A and Beta/Carotene:** These will help in the healing process and in boosting the immune system.
- **Vitamin C and Bioflavonoids:** This combination is healing on the tissues of the body and can increase the function of the immune system.
- **Zinc:** Zinc is very healing for short periods of time. Follow recommendations on the label.

HERBAL REMEDIES

- **Echinacea:** Echinacea is a natural antibiotic effective against viral and bacterial infections.

- **Golden Seal:** This herb is also a natural antibiotic and can help soothe the mucous membranes.
- **Eyebright:** Eyebright can help increase circulation to the eye area. A compress can be made using a tea made from the dried herb and water.
- **Golden Seal, Eyebright and Red Raspberry.** A tea can be made by boiling and straining three to four times. Apply with an eyedropper to the eye area.

CONSTIPATION

Constipation is a condition characterized by a decrease in the number of bowel movements. It occurs when waste progresses too slowly through the intestines. It is also characterized by hard stools which are painful and difficult to pass. It is generally thought that one bowel movement per day is normal among children. And most health professionals feel this is preferable. Some may go a few days without difficulty or others may go three times per day. The real problem is when the stools are hard and difficult to pass.

Infants are another story. Their digestive systems are immature and take time to adjust. Breastfed babies usually have fewer bowel movements than bottle fed babies because the breast milk is used efficiently by the body. As long as the baby appears comfortable, there is no need to worry. As food is introduced into the diet and the baby becomes more active, bowel function will change.

Adequate bowel function is very important. Many health professionals associate many immune related illnesses with constipation. It is felt that toxins from the waste products can accumulate in the bowel and then be reabsorbed into the body, causing problems.

CAUSES

There are a number of factors that can contribute to constipation in children. Among them are lack of exercise, poor diet, lack of fiber, too little liquid, and emotional problems. Some medications can also cause constipation. A physical problem such as an obstruction in the bowel, can also cause constipation. This can be serious and if the child is in severe pain, a medical professional should be consulted. Constipation can lead to other problems such as hemorrhoids, indigestion, heartburn, obesity, varicose veins, hernia, appendicitis, gas and bowel cancer.

HOME CARE

- Increase fiber and liquids in the diet.
- Massaging the lower abdomen may encourage movement.
- Exercise helps keep bowel function regular.
- Have the child sit on the toilet at a regular time each morning to encourage regularity.
- Make meal time relaxing, avoiding stress.
- Enemas can be used in severe cases.

DIETARY GUIDELINES

- Eat regular meals.
- Avoid fatty foods and red meat products, as they are difficult to digest.
- Give the child plenty of pure water each day to drink. At least four glasses per day is recommended.
- Prune juice can help promote bowel function.
- Avoid all junk foods such as soda, chips, french fries, sugar products, and white flour products.

- Add high fiber foods to the diet such as whole grains, pears, apples, oatmeal, bran, grapes and raisins.
- Encourage children to chew their food well before swallowing.
- Herbal laxative teas can be added to fruit juice in small amounts.
- Molasses and warm water can help with constipation.

NUTRITIONAL SUPPLEMENTS

- **Acidophilus and Bifidus:** Acidophilus increases the beneficial bacteria in the digestive tract, helping digestion.
- **B-Complex Vitamins:** They help with the digestive process.
- **Flaxseed Oil:** This helps to soften the stools.
- **Vitamin E:** Vitamin E can help soothe and heal an irritated colon.

HERBAL REMEDIES

- **Aloe Vera:** Aloe Vera juice is a mild laxative.
- **Red Raspberry:** Raspberry tea is mild and soothing on the digestive tract.
- **Licorice:** Licorice tea or extract can help relieve constipation.
- **Cascara Sagrada:** This can be used in small amounts for children for short periods of time.
- **Dandelion:** Dandelion root is a liver tonic and mild laxative.
- **Herbal laxative combinations** can be given to relieve constipation. Some babies are born with poor bowel function.

COUGHS

There are many different types of coughs associated with a variety of conditions. Some are loud while others may be soft, dry, wet, hacking, loose or croupy. If a cough is dry and hacking in nature, it is an indication that an irritant is affecting the respiratory tract. A loose and wet cough is a sign of mucus being produced. Infants and small children will swallow the majority of the mucus which may cause stomach discomfort. Some coughs are wheezing in nature. This could be a sign of asthma or a viral illness of the bronchial tubes. The nature of coughs vary from a slight irritation to a nagging, continuous hacking. A cough usually lasts for only a few days, but it could develop into more serious conditions such as bronchitis, pneumonia or asthma.

A cough is a way of ridding the body of bacteria, viruses, germs, pollen and other irritants. It clears the lungs of foreign material allowing for clear breathing passages. A continuous cough can be irritating and painful for a child. Though it is necessary to cough, it may result in sleeping difficulties, further contributing to the problem.

Some children cough when they are nervous. It may just be a nervous habit. Allergies may also cause a common cough to occur. Allergies can irritate the respiratory tract resulting in a cough.

CAUSES

The respiratory tract becomes inflamed either by a virus or bacteria that causes an increase in the secretions of mucus. A cough accompanied by a fever may be bacterial in nature. A cough may be associated with changes in the seasons. The body may have a delayed reaction as the season begins to change, allowing for the infection to occur. Physical stress on the body such as being over-tired, rundown, recent immunizations, or a growth spurt may result in an illness and cough because of the immune system being compromised. Emotional factors also can result in illnesses such as a cough. New situations, a new baby in the home, negative feelings, problems at school, or changes in the family can all lead to emotional trauma which affect the immune response. When the kidneys and lungs are functioning properly, the lungs will usually remain healthy and not become congested. The skin is an organ of elimination. When exposed to cold weather, the pores close, stopping the skin's ability to eliminate toxins and gases and may send the toxins to the lungs.

HOME CARE

- Avoid exposure to extreme weather changes.
- Use a humidifier in the child's room at night.
- Coughing is a symptom of an illness, so figure out what is causing the problem.

DIETARY GUIDELINES

- When a cough is present, avoid cow's milk products, sugar, peanuts, or any foods with an allergic response or that are mucus forming.
- Offer plenty of fluids such as juices, soups, and herbal teas. Avoid cold drinks.
- Citrus juices contain vitamin C which is healing.

NUTRITIONAL SUPPLEMENTS

- **Vitamin C:** Vitamin C helps in preventing illness, reducing inflammation and in stimulating the immune system. It can help soothe the throat.

- **Vitamin A and Beta-Carotene:** They help stimulate the immune system and aid in the healing process.

HERBAL REMEDIES

- **Lobelia:** Lobelia is useful in calming the cough, reducing inflammation, and removing obstructions from the body. An extract form can be used. A small amount is recommended; one drop under the tongue. Lobelia extract can also be rubbed on the spine to help relax the muscles.
- **Echinacea:** It helps heal and prevent infection. Echinacea is also useful for reducing mucus.
- **Licorice:** Licorice contains antibacterial properties. It can be given as a tea to soothe the throat helping to control a cough. It has a sweet flavor which is helpful when administering to children.
- **Marshmallow:** Marshmallow helps reduce inflammation and soothe the throat.
- **Mullein:** Mullein is useful on the respiratory tract.
- **Ginger:** Ginger helps in warming the system which stimulates the body's immune system to combat the illness.
- **Horehound:** Horehound helps in clearing congestion from the lungs.
- **Garlic:** Garlic is a natural antibiotic which can help heal.
- **Peppermint:** Peppermint tea with fresh lemon or lime juice can help with coughs.
- **Herbal cough extracts** can help which contain Fenugreek, Comfrey, Yerba Santa, Hyssop and Wild Cherry.

CRADLE CAP

Cradle cap is a condition which forms a scaly crust on the top of an infant's scalp but can also occur on the eyebrows, eyelids, on the sides of the nose and behind the ears. It is quite common in babies between the ages of two weeks and a year. It is a form of seborrheic dermatitis which is an inflammatory condition of the skin. It is characterized by scaly crusts white or yellowish in color and oval or roundish shape. It is similar to dandruff but the scales are greasy.

The baby's head should be washed and scrubbed daily to prevent the condition from worsening. But washing daily will not prevent the condition from occurring. A gentle brush specifically for babies can help clear some of the crusts from the scalp.

CAUSES

Cradle cap is caused by overactive sebaceous glands. They secrete oil that dries and forms a yellowish crust. This crusting can plug the glands which in turn secrete more oil in trying to unplug the glands. Sensitive skin may also contribute to the problem as well as insufficient stimulation to the scalp.

Home Care

- Wash the infant's scalp daily, using a soft brush.

DIETARY GUIDELINES

- If nursing, eliminate refined sugar and white flour products. They contribute to the growth of bacteria and yeast.
- A healthy diet is important when breast feeding. Eat plenty of whole foods emphasizing vegetables and fruits.

NUTRITIONAL SUPPLEMENTS

- **Acidophilus and Bifidus:** Acidophilus helps improve the healthy, beneficial bacteria needed in the body. When nursing, the mother can take a supplement. Bottle fed babies can take it in the bottle with formula. (1/8 t. per day)
- **Multi-Vitamin/Mineral Supplement:** Nursing mothers should take a supplement. Infants can take a supplement designed for their age and needs.
- **Olive Oil:** Warm olive oil can be applied to the baby's scalp and left overnight. Wash with a mild shampoo to remove the scales the next morning.
- **Almond Oil/Vitamin E:** These can also be applied to the scalp and left for 20 minutes. Then wash and remove scales.

HERBAL REMEDIES

- **Tea Tree Oil Shampoo:** This can be used in a diluted form. Make sure and protect the baby's eyes.
- **Aloe Vera:** Aloe Vera liquid can be applied to the scalp before washing the hair.
- **Evening Primrose Oil:** Massage Evening Primrose oil into the baby's scalp at bedtime and wash in the morning.

CROUP

Croup can be a frightening condition for both the child and the parent. It is an infection of the upper respiratory tract that causes constriction and narrowing of the larynx and trachea. It is most often viral in nature. Inflammation in the voice box and windpipe causes swelling and difficulty in breathing and talking, resulting in a brassy, bark-like cough. There is also a wheezing with the intake of air. The condition can be mild or severe. Respiration usually appears to be shallow and rapid with the abdominal muscles pulling in as a breath is taken.

It is a common condition most often affecting children from age three months to four years. The condition usually worsens at night. And croup, as with many viral infections, commonly occurs in the late fall and winter.

Humidifying the air can help. Taking the child out into the cold air can temporarily relieve the problem. The child will probably prefer to sleep in a slightly upright position.

CAUSES

Croup is most often caused by a virus, but some serious cases may be bacterial in nature. Congestion and mucus may dry in the throat area causing difficulty in breathing. Croup can also be caused by a cold virus settling in the upper respiratory tract. Cases of croup have been linked to allergies, air pollution and milk products.

HOME CARE

• Use a cool mist humidifier in the child's room.
• A cool compress to the throat may control an attack.
• Remain calm and reassuring to the child.

- Bundle the child in a blanket and take them outside for a few minutes if it is a cool night.
- Have the child sleep in a slightly upright position.
- Keep the child away from cigarette smoke.
- Apply hot onion packs over the chest and back.

DIETARY GUIDELINES

- Avoid dairy products and mucus forming foods.
- Give children ample liquids such as citrus juices, herbal teas, and warm vegetable broth. This helps to loosen the mucus.

NUTRITIONAL SUPPLEMENTS

- **Vitamin C and Bioflavonoids:** This combination helps with healing and strengthening the immune system.
- **Vitamin A:** Vitamin A is healing on the mucous membranes.
- **Vitamin E:** It helps the immune system and aids in tissue repair.
- **Zinc:** Zinc lozenges can be used to suck on for short periods of time. They help with healing and immune function as well as soothe the throat.

HERBAL REMEDIES

- **Ginger:** Ginger as a tea or a Ginger bath can help to encourage sweating and promote healing.
- **Garlic/Onion:** An old remedy suggests placing sliced onions and garlic between warm sterile cloths and placing on the chest area. This can help open the congested areas. Garlic can be taken in extract form to heal and prevent infection.

- **Eucalyptus:** The oil can be rubbed on the chest area in a diluted form for children.
- **Marshmallow:** Marshmallow helps to soothe the inflamed areas.
- **Hyssop:** This helps as an expectorant and to quiet the cough.
- **Wild Cherry:** This works as a cough suppressant.
- **Licorice:** Licorice can help soothe the inflamed areas and heal.
- **Mullein:** This helps to control a cough.
- **Comfrey/Fenugreek:** These are useful in healing the mucous membranes and the respiratory tract.
- **Lobelia:** A small amount under the tongue can help control coughing and clear mucus congestion.
- **Herbal laxatives** can help relieve constipation if it is a problem.

CUTS AND ABRASIONS

Cuts and abrasions are a part of childhood. Skinned knees and hands will occur when children are allowed to play and explore the outdoors. Injuries should be treated because of the possibility of infection. Young children are more vulnerable to infection because they have not yet acquired all the antibodies to fight infection. Some areas, such as the head, mouth, facial area, hands and feet, have blood vessels close to the skin's surface which causes them to bleed more.

Most cuts can be treated at home. But if the bleeding is profuse and the wound appears to be gaping, medical attention should be sought, as stitches may be necessary.

Stop the bleeding by applying direct pressure with a clean cloth to the affected area. Once the bleeding has stopped, clean the area with soap, water and apply a disinfectant. Cover with a bandage or gauze.

CAUSES

Injuries, such as cuts and abrasions, can be caused by a myriad of things. When learning to ride a bike, a child will no doubt sustain numerous cuts and scrapes. Climbing, jumping and just walking can all lead to injury. Caution children to be careful and avoid hazardous situations.

HOME CARE

- Stop the bleeding by applying direct pressure.
- Cleanse the area with a mild soap and water.
- Apply a sterile gauze or bandage to the wound.

DIETARY GUIDELINES

- Avoid refined sugars as they slow the healing process.
- Encourage whole, natural foods, vegetables and fruits which strengthen the immune system.

NUTRITIONAL SUPPLEMENTS

- **Vitamin A and Beta-Carotene:** These are healing and soothing on tissues of the body.
- **Vitamin C and Bioflavonoids:** These work to speed healing, reduce inflammation and in strengthening the immune system.
- **Honey:** Honey can be applied to an injury. It aids in healing and contains natural antibiotic properties according to an article in *Lancet,* January 9, 1993 page 341.

HERBAL REMEDIES

- **Aloe Vera:** Aloe Vera can be applied to the wound to speed healing and reduce scarring.
- **Echinacea:** Echinacea is a natural antibiotic to aid in healing and preventing infection.
- **Golden Seal:** This helps with both viral and bacterial infections and can help speed healing.
- **Calendula:** It contains antibacterial properties, soothes the skin and speeds healing.

DEHYDRATION

Dehydration in infants and children can be a serious condition. They become dehydrated more easily than adults because of their greater need for fluids. If body fluids are lost, a child can easily become listless and unresponsive. Some signs of dehydration are shallow breathing, sunken eyes, weakness, dry mouth, and a rapid pulse. With a loss of fluids, the blood volume is less, which can result in a fall in blood pressure. This must be corrected quickly or medical attention should be given.

CAUSES

Dehydration can be caused by diarrhea, vomiting, excess perspiration from the heat or a high fever. A child will probably be thirsty but may not be able to keep anything down. An infant may not show any signs other than being ill. Watch the baby to see if less urine is being passed than usual. This can be a serious condition if not treated. Fluids should be administered promptly and if the child does not respond or keep the fluids down, a medical professional should be seen.

HOME CARE

- If dehydration is suspected, administer fluids quickly, a sip at a time, to avoid vomiting.
- If the child will not drink, seek medical attention to avoid serious complications.

DIETARY GUIDELINES

- Administer fluids as soon as possible.
- Fluids which contain minerals and salts in correct proportions should be given to provide adequate electrolyte balance. Rehydration fluids are available in drugstores.
- A home remedy includes 4 cups boiled water, 3 T. honey, 1/4 t. natural sea salt, 1/4 t. baking soda. Give sips to avoid vomiting. Orange juice can be given, alternating this solution.
- Brown rice water will help replenish nutrients.

NATURAL SUPPLEMENTS

- Vitamin and mineral supplements should be given only after the child is feeling better and can keep foods down.

HERBAL REMEDIES

- **Ginger:** Ginger tea can help replenish the body when dehydration occurs and aid in digestion.
- **Peppermint:** Peppermint tea can be soothing, especially after vomiting.

DIAPER RASH

Diaper rash is a common problem with infants in diapers. Most babies have some problems with diaper rash at times. The skin around the diaper area becomes inflamed, red, rough and bumps sometimes are present. Nine to twelve month olds are most commonly affected. The diaper area should be kept clean, warm and dry. A child can be allowed to go without a diaper to let the area dry out and breathe.

CAUSES

Diaper rash is usually caused by contact with feces, urine, detergents and chemicals. If a child is left in a soiled diaper for too long, they will be more susceptible to getting a rash. Children have tender skin and a dirty diaper should be changed as quickly as possible. Some believe that disposable diapers have contributed to the problem and that cloth diapers are less apt to contribute to diaper rash. Others feel just the opposite. Regardless of the parent's preference, a dirty diaper needs attention. Too much uric acid in the urine can contribute. Make sure the baby drinks plenty of pure water to dilute the urine. Diarrhea and antibiotics can also make the skin more vulnerable to a rash.

HOME CARE

- Keep the diaper area clean and change soiled diapers promptly.
- Let the child go without a diaper and expose to the sunlight if possible.
- Apply a mixture of 1 T. baking soda and 4 ounces pure water to the diaper area after cleaning. This can help make the area more alkaline, counteracting the acidity of urine

and stools.
- Apply cornstarch to the dry area.

DIETARY GUIDELINES

- The baby or child should be given a lot of pure water. This can help dilute acidic urine which may contribute to the problem. Nursing mothers should also drink plenty of pure water.
- Nursing mothers should eliminate foods from their diet which may be contributing to the problem such as milk products, yeast foods, sugar, and caffeine.
- The introduction of new foods in the baby's diet may cause problems. Be careful in choosing foods and eliminate if a problem is suspected.

NUTRITIONAL SUPPLEMENTS

- **Acidophilus and Bifidus:** Acidophilus can help especially if the problems is related to a yeast infection. A baby can take 1/8 t. in their bottle. A nursing mother can also benefit by taking the recommend dosage.
- **Vitamin E:** Vitamin E is healing and can be applied to the affected area.
- **Zinc Oxide:** This can help speed the healing process.

HERBAL REMEDIES

- **Aloe Vera:** Aloe Vera is healing and soothing when applied to the area.
- **Calendula:** Apply in a lotion or in a warm bath to soothe and heal.

- **Comfrey:** An ointment with Comfrey can help soothe and heal.
- **Evenining Primrose:** A lotion or extract can help reduce inflammation.

DIARRHEA

Diarrhea is a condition commonly occurring in infants and young children. It is characterized by frequent, loose stools and cramping. It is not considered a disorder in itself but a symptom of another physiological condition. This is one way in which the body attempts to eliminate toxins, viruses, germs and other irritations. It is not usually a severe disorder and corrects itself within a few days. Medications given to treat the diarrhea may inhibit the body from performing its natural function. But consideration should be taken if the condition persists. Infants and small children can become dehydrated quickly if the diarrhea is persistent. Breastfed babies generally have loose stools. This is not considered diarrhea. Children have different patterns of bowel movements and what is normal for one may not be normal for another. Chronic diarrhea may be the sign of a more serious intestinal problem.

CAUSES

Acute diarrhea in children is usually due to feeding habits. Infants may be overfed when parents use this to soothe a fussy baby. Food poisoning can also cause diarrhea. Properly storing and preparation of food is extremely important when small children are involved.

Chronic diarrhea can be caused by a variety of factors. Viruses can enter the intestinal tract causing irritation and inflammation. This leads to the secretion of excess fluids causing cramps and diarrhea. Allergies to foods such as cow's milk may lead to chronic diarrhea. Other common allergic foods include eggs, chicken, nuts, and wheat. If the condition persists, the diet of the child should be considered.

Some individuals feel that some cases of diarrhea are actually related to constipation when the intestinal tract is so badly clogged that the fecal solids are being held back and only the eliminative liquids are allowed to pass.

Some children have sensitive intestinal tracts and may have diarrhea with any infectious condition. It may occur when the body is attempting to rid itself of toxins. Medications are also a concern. Some antibiotics can cause diarrhea as well as over-the-counter drugs.

HOME CARE

- Watch for signs of dehydration.
- If there is blood in the stools, seek medical attention.
- Give adequate fluid to replace the fluid lost.
- Ice chips may be easier to keep down when the child has an upset stomach.

DIETARY GUIDELINES

- Dehydration is the first concern with infants and small children. Give the child frequent sips of water or clear liquid. Don't offer too much, as vomiting may result.
- A fluid replacement drink can be offered when the child begins to feel better. 1/2 teaspoon of honey and a pinch of salt in 8 ounces of clear fruit juice or water can be used.
- Avoid medications, if possible, to treat the condition.
- Avoid dairy products or other foods which may cause allergies.

- Nursing can continue during bouts with diarrhea. The mother can add acidophilus to her diet.
- Introduce foods gradually to the diet. A simple diet with foods that are easy to digest should be given first.
- Refined sugars can aggravate the condition, especially if the diarrhea is caused by bacteria which thrive on the sugar.
- Rice or barley water can be given to infants.
- Carrot soup is an old home remedy to help diarrhea.
- Papaya juice is healing and soothing on the intestinal tract.
- Bananas can help to relieve diarrhea.
- Brown rice water can offer nutrients and help with diarrhea.
- A high fiber diet is important to regulate bowel function.

NUTRITIONAL SUPPLEMENTS

- **Potassium:** Potassium can be lost when diarrhea is present. A supplement may be beneficial.
- **Acidophilus and Bifidus:** Replacing the friendly bacteria helps restore healthy flora in the intestines.
- **Carob Powder:** This helps to normalize bowel function.

HERBAL REMEDIES

- **Slippery Elm:** Slippery Elm is healing and soothing to the intestines. Powdered forms can be added to applesauce or juice and given to children over three years of age.
- **Red Raspberry:** Red Raspberry can be given in tea form. It is a mild treatment for diarrhea.
- **Golden Seal:** Golden Seal contains antibiotic properties which can control forms of bacterial diarrhea. It contains berberine which helps to control acute diarrhea from bacterial infections.

- **Dill:** Dill helps inhibit the growth of intestinal bacteria.
- **Ginger:** A weak Ginger tea can help settle the stomach and soothe the intestinal tract.
- **Catnip:** Catnip tea is mild and beneficial for diarrhea in children.
- **Marshmallow:** Marshmallow is soothing and healing on the intestinal tract and mucus membranes.
- **Bowel combinations** can help heal chronic conditions and strengthen the intestinal tract.

DYSLEXIA

Dyslexia is a common problem in children, and it is estimated that one in ten children suffer from some form of dyslexia. It is a term used to describe children who have difficulties with reading and writing. They may see things backwards, have coordination difficulties and have trouble identifying shapes. Dyslexic children may be late in crawling, walking and talking. Some may completely miss the crawling stage. A dyslexic child may have problems with hearing and eyesight.

Some of the signs of dyslexia may include: words used wrong, writing backwards, difficulty relating sounds to letters, reversing letters, dropping part of syllables in words, memory problems, difficulties following left to right and frustration because of learning difficulties.

CAUSES

Dyslexia is thought to be a disorganization problem in the central nervous system. It is seen as a left brain dysfunction. The signals seem to get mixed up during the electrical transmission of information from the left side of the brain.

Eighty percent of dyslexics are male and some think a male hormone imbalance may be involved. The problem is not related to retardation, as the difficulties are in reading and writing and not the thinking process.

HOME CARE

- Watch for signals as the child enters school.
- Have the eyes and ears checked for problems.
- Be patient and understanding. The dyslexic child will require more time and energy to learn.
- Help them build a good self esteem in spite of the learning problems by emphasizing their good qualities.
- A chiropractor may be able to help with dyslexia if they have experience in the area.
- Test for allergies, as they may be related.

DIETARY GUIDELINES

- Avoid sugar, refined foods, chocolate, wheat, and other stress foods.
- Eat a high fiber diet.
- Eat fruits, vegetables, whole grains, brown rice, millet, buckwheat, oats and rye.
- Avoid foods with hormone additives such as beef, chicken, pork, eggs, and dairy products. Eat hormone free foods.

NUTRITIONAL SUPPLEMENTS

- **Multi-Vitamin and Mineral Supplement:** This can help ensure adequate amounts of nutrients for health. Proper nutrition is an advantage in the learning process.

- **B-Complex:** The B-Complex vitamins can help strengthen the nervous system and improve brain function.
- **Vitamin C and Bioflavonoids:** This combination helps the immune system and in healing.
- **Vitamin E:** Vitamin E is useful for hormone balance.
- **Calcium and Magnesium:** These help to build the central nervous system.
- **Chlorophyll/Blue-Green Algae:** These help to nourish the blood and brain.
- **Amino Acid Supplement:** Amino acids help to strengthen the nervous system.

HERBAL REMEDIES

- **Bee Pollen:** Bee Pollen is rich in protein, vitamins, minerals and enzymes and is very nutritious and helpful in brain function.
- **Chamomile:** This helps to soothe and relax the nerves.
- **Ginkgo:** Ginkgo increases the blood flow to the brain and helps improve memory.
- **Gotu Kola:** This is food for the brain and helps to build the nerves and increase memory.
- **Hops:** Hops is a nervine herb to help calm the nerves.
- **Passion Flower:** This helps to support and strengthen the immune system to calm and relax.
- **Scullcap:** Scullcap is a nervine herb to help with restlessness.

EARACHE

Millions of children are treated each year for middle ear infections (otitis media). Seventy percent of all children are known to have suffered from ear infections during their childhood. This conditions is most commonly found in children between the ages of six months and three years. This is a very painful condition, causing discomfort and loss of sleep for children and their parents. This is the most common childhood disorder. But most children will outgrow the problem by the time they reach three years of age.

The ear consists of the outer, middle and inner ears. The outer is the visible part that extends from the side of the head. The middle ear involves three small bones which are responsible for carrying the sound vibrations to the inner ear. The inner ear with nerve endings makes the hearing process complete and helps maintain balance.

CAUSES

The most common type of ear infection involves the middle ear. It is connected to the sinuses and throat by the eustachian tube. Fluid from the tube can drain through the nose and throat under normal conditions. But when the eustachian tube is blocked, pain and infection may result. Infants and small children have small eustachian tubes which can easily become blocked. The tube is often more horizontal than vertical, allowing for fluid buildup. This fluid offers an environment for bacteria to grow. As children grow, the structure of the inner ear changes which helps the fluid to drain properly, avoiding infection. Ear infections often accompany colds and respiratory problems.

Ear infections are usually caused by two organisms known as *Streptococcus pneumonia* and the *Hemophilus influenza*. Viral infections may occasionally cause earaches. Weak tissue support in the eustachian tube and abnormal openings in the tube can cause fluid to build up, leading to infections. Allergies are also considered a factor in ear infections.

Tala Nsouli, an allergist at Georgetown University School of Medicine, became concerned when he realized that many of the patients he treated for allergies suffered from chronic ear infections and even hearing loss. He did a study with his colleagues testing 104 children ranging in age from 18 months to nine years who had suffered from ear infections over a three month period or had repeated episodes over a period of five months. Eighty-one of those children tested positive to allergies, mainly to wheat and milk. For four months these children were taken off the foods that caused the allergic reactions. Seventy of them got better when kept off the offending foods. After the four month period, the foods were gradually introduced back into the children's diets. Sixty-six of those children got ear infections again. This is certainly strong evidence linking ear infections and allergies, and parents should take note and check into the possibility if their children suffer from recurring ear infections.

Bottle fed infants are more likely to develop ear infections. This may be the result of two contributing factors. One is an allergic reaction to the formula. Another factor may be the position of the infant when fed a bottle allowing for the fluid to stay in the tube.

Swimmer's ear occurs when the fluid is trapped in the ear canal. An infection may occur. This is common in children who spend a lot of time at the swimming pool.

The usual treatment involves antibiotics. Many doctors and parents fear hearing loss may occur if the condition is not treated immediately. For this reason, many children are put on antibiotics for extended periods of time because the ear infections recur and persist. Dr. Robert Mendelsohn discusses some of his experiences in his book *How To Raise A Healthy Child...In Spite Of Your Doctor.* "The only case in which the use of antibiotics can remotely be justified is if the ear is actually discharging pus, which occurs in less than 1 percent of ear infections, and I'm not convinced that it can be justified even then."

A series of controlled studies have revealed that the use of antibiotics for treatment of ear infections makes no difference in terms of the important outcomes—hearing loss, spread of infection, or mastoiditis. Their use may slightly shorten the duration of pain and infection, but the trade-off is that the antibiotics also reduce the body's natural immune response. Consequently, in order to slightly reduce the duration of the infection, you increase the possibility that the child will have new infections every four to six weeks." Tubes, myringotomy, may be inserted through the eardrums to increase the fluid drainage. This treatment is controversial and may actually increase the risk of ear infection.

Whether to use antibiotics or not is up to the individual. But more people are looking at the statistics and results of recent research before making a decision as to the best path to take when dealing with earaches and infections.

HOME CARE

- Do not use any eardrops if the eardrum has ruptured.
- Prop the child at a 30 degree angle to promote drainage to reduce the pain.
- A warm compress can help reduce the pain.

DIETARY GUIDELINES

- Avoid any foods which may cause allergies such as dairy and wheat.
- Fresh juices are recommended as they help to dilute mucus secretions.

- Liquids are important such as pure water, herbal teas and clear soups.

NUTRITIONAL SUPPLEMENTS

- **Vitamin A and Beta-Carotene:** These are healing and help with infections.
- **Vitamin C and Bioflavonoids:** This helps in increasing immunity, reduce inflammation, and in healing the capillaries.
- **Zinc:** Zinc helps boost the immune system and reduce the chance of infection. Lozenges can be given on a short term basis.
- **Manganese:** Studies have found manganese deficiencies to be linked to incidence of ear infections.
- **Acidophilus and Bifidus:** This is especially important for children taking antibiotics, as it helps to restore the beneficial bacteria.
- **Indoles:** Dietary indoles can help strengthen the immune system. They are found in some children's combination supplements.

HERBAL REMEDIES

- **Echinacea:** This is a natural antibiotic to help fight infection and build immunity. It should not be used for extended periods of time.
- **Garlic:** A few drops of warm garlic oil can be placed in the ear if the eardrum has not ruptured. Nothing should be put in the ear if the eardrum has burst. Garlic pills and capsules can also be taken to increase immunity and to speed healing.
- **Lobelia:** Lobelia is relaxing and helps clear obstructions. A drop can be placed in the ear if the eardrum is intact.

- **Passion Flower:** This helps relax the child and relieve pain.
- **Fenugreek:** Fenugreek helps to remove mucus and promote drainage.
- **Mullein:** The oil warmed is an old remedy to reduce inflammation and pain.
- **St. John's Wort:** The oil can be warmed and applied to the ear for pain and healing.

ECZEMA

Eczema is a chronic skin disorder characterized by inflammation of the skin, flaking skin, redness, oozing and extreme itching. This condition is also known as dermatitis. The skin cells can become thick and discolored over a period of time. The itching can become so severe that a child will most likely scratch, preferring the pain and bleeding to the itching. The area can become infected and weeping will result.

In a small child, the first signs of the condition may be red, chapped cheeks. The most common areas where eczema is seen are the face, scalp, behind the ears, elbow creases, knees and groin area. Tiny pimples may appear on a child's buttocks as well. The condition can spread over a period of time, clear up and recur.

Eczema is a condition that can occur at any age. It is most commonly found in young girls. Fifty percent of infants with eczema outgrow it by the age of eighteen months. It can be either acute or chronic, lasting for years with periods of remission and reccurrence of the condition.

Atopic dermatitis is a type of eczema that appears in infants usually around two to three months of age. It is considered an allergic type and often found in other family members. Foods, pollen, dust, or other allergens can induce an outbreak.

Contact dermatitis is the more common of the two types of eczema. An infant may break out from drooling or licking the lips. It may occur from foods, contact with certain toxins, chemicals, detergents, cosmetics, wool, or environmental pollutants. It is found most often in older children. The skin is very sensitive to irritants and any numerous items can cause a reaction.

CAUSES

Allergies are associated with both types of eczema. It is thought to be hereditary and two-thirds of individuals suffering from eczema have other family member with the disorder. Different factors thought to trigger a reaction are stress, food allergies, sweating, detergents, chemicals, wool, or environmental pollutants. Studies done point to food allergies as a leading cause of eczema. For infants, the most likely allergen would be cow's milk. Children and adults may be sensitive to dairy products and grains. Some believe that congested colon and kidneys can contribute to skin diseases, and this should be considered with skin conditions.

HOME CARE

- Keep the child's fingernails trimmed to avoid scratching.
- Use only very mild soaps to cleanse the area. Soap can be very drying and adds to the problems with eczema.
- Wool, silk and synthetic fabrics may irritate the skin.
- Expose the skin to fresh air and moderate amounts of sunlight as this may help with healing.
- Cotton clothing should be worn by the child as it is more comfortable and less irritating on the skin.
- Avoid overdressing the child as this can cause sweating and irritate the eczema.
- Avoid foods and irritants that may cause allergies. Some detergents can be very irritating.

DIETARY GUIDELINES

- Wait to introduce foods such as citrus fruits, cow's milk and wheat until the child is at least a year old. These may make a child more susceptible to allergy-related disorders.
- Use an elimination diet to look for possible foods causing problems. If breastfeeding, the mother should do the same.
- Encourage foods such as cooked carrots, green leafy vegetables, celery, grapes, papaya and pears.
- Make vegetable soup and use a healthy diet.

NUTRITIONAL SUPPLEMENTS

- **Essential Fatty Acids:** Some studies point to a deficiency in the essential fatty acids in individuals suffering from eczema. Flaxseed oil, black current oil and evening primrose oil are some suggestions.
- **Vitamin A and Beta-Carotene:** They both promote healing and help in the development and functioning of the skin.
- **Vitamin C and Bioflavonoids:** They help with healing and in reducing inflammation.
- **Vitamin E:** Vitamin E is beneficial on the skin for healing and soothing. It can be taken internally or applied directly to the affected area.
- **Zinc:** Zinc aids in the healing process and has been used successfully in treating those suffering from eczema. Follow directions on the label.

HERBAL REMEDIES

- **Chaparral:** A bath with Chaparral tea can help soothe the skin, promote healing and reduce itching.
- **Echinacea:** An Echinacea tincture taken internally helps

prevent infection, boost the immune system, promote healing, and purify the blood.

- **Burdock:** Burdock root can be given in tea form to help cleanse the blood and heal the skin. It has a long history of use in treating eczema.
- **St. John's Wort:** This has been used as an oil traditionally to treat skin disorders.
- **Red Clover:** Red Clover is a well known blood purifier useful in treating skin disorders.
- **Licorice:** Licorice is an anti-inflammatory and helps in reducing the secretions of histamine. Ointments containing Licorice may be helpful.
- **Cascara Sagrada:** This can help with clearing toxins from the body through the bowels and working to relieve constipation which may be a contributing factor.
- **Aloe Vera:** Aloe Vera is soothing on the skin and healing.
- **Herbal combinations** for the bowels and kidneys may help with skin disorders.

FEVER

A fever is a symptom of an illness. It is characterized by the temperature elevating at least one degree above the norm which is 98.6 degrees F. or 37 degrees C. Children's temperatures will vary, depending on clothing worn, level of activity or the time of day.

An elevated body temperature is a reaction of the immune system in attempting to destroy bacteria and viruses that enter the body. Some viruses and bacteria falter in the body when the temperature is elevated. It should not always be considered negative, as it is a way of fighting infection. A fever also causes an increase in production of the white blood cells as well as their speed of response.

The exact temperature of a child may not always indicate

how sick they really are. A child with a mild virus may have a 104 degree F. fever while another with pneumonia may have a 101 degree F. fever. The important thing to do is to watch how a child acts. If they still are active, it is probably a mild condition. A fever may precede conditions such as measles, chickenpox and roseola in babies. A child with a high fever will generally feel lousy. But when the fever is brought down, a child with a mild cold or virus will feel better while the one suffering from a more serious condition will probably continue to feel badly.

A fever over 102 degrees F. in a child should probably be treated. Medical attention should be sought if there are any serious concerns as to the child's condition.

A febrile seizure may accompany a fever in some children. It is characterized by jerking, shaking, eyes rolling back, listlessness and confusion. There are no harmful side effects or answers as to why some children are predisposed to febrile seizures. They usually accompanying a high fever and are frightening to see. Though there are thought to be no harmful side effects from the seizures, a child should be seen by a physician after a seizure occurs to rule out other problems.

CAUSES

A fever usually accompanies a viral or bacterial infection. Some common conditions often seen with a fever are colds, flu, sore throat, tonsillitis, earaches and infections, diarrhea, urinary tract infections, roseola, chickenpox, measles, pneumonia and meningitis. A fever may also be caused from conditions such as sunburn, dehydration, bee stings, allergic reactions and overexertion.

When some conditions are present in the body, it causes proteins known as pyrogens to be released, acting on the section of brain which controls body temperature.

159

HOME CARE

- Some health care professionals believe that a mild fever, under 100 degrees, should not be suppressed. Taking fever reducing medications may slow the recovery process.
- Warm water should be used when trying to bring down a fever. Cold water can bring the fever down too quickly, producing chills.
- Sponge the body with a wash cloth.
- Encourage the child to rest.
- Be careful not to overdress a child or infant.
- Fluids should be offered to avoid dehydration.
- A cool cloth applied to the forehead can help lower a fever.
- Make sure the feet are kept warm.

DIETARY GUIDELINES

- Dehydration is a concern with a fever. Encourage ample amounts of fluids such as pure water, popsicles, herbal teas, soups, and diluted fruit juices.
- Mild foods such as yogurt, fruits and vegetables are recommended.
- Do not force foods if the child refuses, but do encourage fluids.

NUTRITIONAL SUPPLEMENTS

- **Vitamin C and Bioflavonoids:** Vitamin C can help heal infections and has anti-inflammatory properties. It helps reduce fevers and helps in eliminating toxins from the body. A powder form may be added to liquids.
- **Vitamin A:** Vitamin A helps in healing, fighting infection and in boosting the immune system.

- **Indoles:** Dietary indoles can help strengthen the immune system to fight disease.

HERBAL REMEDIES

- **Raspberry:** Raspberry tea is useful in treating childhood illnesses and in reducing fever.
- **Echinacea:** This can help fight infection and promote healing.
- **Golden Seal:** Golden Seal helps boost the immune system and aids in fighting infection.
- **Lobelia:** A small drop of the extract can help reduce a fever.
- **Ginger:** Ginger tea helps with fevers, colds, and stomach problems.
- **Catnip:** Catnip tea can help soothe and lower fevers.

FLATULENCE

Flatulence is also known as passing gas or breaking wind. It is a common everyday occurrence which usually doesn't cause any serious concerns. Most children experience flatulence from time to time. Stomach gas is often associated with colic in babies, especially those bottle fed, but can be alleviated by gently burping. Gas can cause temporary pain at times.

CAUSES

Bottle fed babies are more prone to flatulence which may be painful and cause problems with colic. Swallowing air with the formula may cause gas to accumulate in the stomach.

Make sure the nipple size is correct and that the holes in the bottle are not too large or too small.

Food intolerance can also cause gas pains. The baby may have food allergies, especially to cow's milk. Some formulas may not be tolerated well by infants. Even breast fed babies may suffer from this problem due to the dairy intake of the mother. Children are especially sensitive to food allergies and lactose intolerance. One symptom may be flatulence.

An abnormal bacterial flora in the intestines can also lead to flatulence. This may occur because of antibiotic therapy, improper digestion, or a weakened immune system. Chronic problems may need a medical doctor's assistance to determine the source of the flatulence.

HOME CARE

- Check for food sensitivities.
- Avoid foods that may cause problems.
- Make sure the child is not constipated.
- Ensure a healthy diet.

DIETARY GUIDELINES

- Avoid dairy products, especially for infants, as this can lead to an intolerance and flatulence.
- Encourage a diet rich in whole grains and vegetables.
- A low fat diet is easier to digest.
- Avoid all foods commonly associated with allergies such as wheat, chocolate, raisins, cabbage, broccoli, cheese, and sugar.
- Encourage a lot of fluids such as pure water, fruit juices, and vegetable juices.
- Foods which help prevent flatulence include fruit juices, peas, carrots, beets, potatoes, stewed fruits, eggs, chicken, fish, oatmeal, and creamed wheat.

Nutritional Supplements

- **Acidophilus and Bifidus:** This can help normalize the intestinal flora and improve digestion.
- **Carob Powder:** This can help improve the bowel function.

Herbal Remedies

- **Chamomile:** Chamomile tea can be given to children and in a diluted form to infants. It is soothing and healing on the stomach.
- **Raspberry:** Raspberry tea is soothing on the stomach and intestines.
- **Ginger:** A weak Ginger tea can help the stomach and relieve gas pains.

HAYFEVER (See Allergies)

HEAD INJURIES

Most head injuries are not serious and result from a fall or blow to the head. If a child seems dazed, listless, in severe pain, has blurred speech, bleeds form the ear, nose or mouth, or vomits, medical attention should be given to the child. Internal bleeding may cause problems to appear during the first few hours after an injury occurs. Keep the child under observation for a while after suffering a head injury. Minor head injuries may be accompanied by a headache.

More serious head injuries may result in dilated pupils, drowsiness, confusion, loss of consciousness, concussion, severe pain, uncoordination, paralysis, or convulsions. Some may also cause a loss of memory which is usually temporary. If any of these symptoms are seen in the child, seek medical attention immediately as bleeding in the brain may have occurred.

CAUSES

Head injuries are usually caused by a fall or blow to the head. Automobile accidents are one of the leading causes of head injuries in children. Always use child safety seats and seatbelts for older children whenever traveling by car. When children are riding bikes, roller blading, skiing or playing hockey, have them wear helmets to prevent injury to the brain.

HOME CARE

- Keep the child still and observe for an hour after an injury occurs.   ·
- Teach a child to protect himself and to be cautious when playing.
- Keep a child awake for a few hours after an injury.

DIETARY GUIDELINES

- Do not feed a child right after an injury.
- Liquids can be given if desired.

NUTRITIONAL SUPPLEMENTS

- **Vitamin E:** It helps increase the oxygen to the brain.
- **Vitamin A and Beta-Carotene:** These are healing on the tissues and help strengthen the immune system.

Herbal Remedies

- **Gotu Kola:** This is useful to promote brain function such as memory and thinking skills.
- **Capsicum:** This can help stimulate circulation and brain function.
- **Ginkgo:** Ginkgo is useful for brain function.
- **A nervous system combination** can be healing to the brain.

HEAD LICE

Head lice are passed from child to child, usually in a day care or school environment. Head lice are tiny insects that thrive on the scalp. They are spread by direct contact most often between children. Children sharing hats, or working closely, can pass the lice. The lice look like tiny lumps of scalp and the eggs (nits) can be seen attached to the hair shaft. The female lice continue laying eggs each day and must be stopped to prevent further infestation. The lice cause itching on the scalp.

Causes

Head lice is not related to hygiene as some might think. It is passed from child to child by direct contact. And head lice show no preference between socio-economic groups. All children who attend public school, play with friends, go to day care, attend camp, or associate with other children are at risk.

Dr. Henry Lindlar says in his book *Nature's Cure,* "Head lice and similar parasites peculiar to other parts of the body live on scrofulous and psoric toxins. These pests do not remain with all people who have been exposed to them, but only those whose internal or external filth conditions furnish the parasites with the means of sustenance."

HOME CARE

- Examine the scalp using a flashlight if necessary to check for infestation.
- Use a fine-toothed comb to rid the scalp of lice.
- Wash all bedding, clothing, towels, and hats in hot water.

DIETARY GUIDELINES

- Avoid sugar products as this may encourage infestation.
- Encourage healthy, whole, nutritious foods.

NUTRITIONAL SUPPLEMENTS

- **Vitamin C and Bioflavonoids:** These work together to speed healing and improve the function of the immune system.
- **Vitamin A and Beta-Carotene:** These are healing and aid the immune system.

HERBAL REMEDIES

- **Eucalyptus, Pennyroyal, Rosemary, Olive Oil:** Combine 1/2 teaspoon of Eucalyptus, Pennyroyal, and Rosemary. Add 2 1/2 tablespoons of olive oil. If it burns the skin, add more olive oil to the liquid. Wash the child's scalp with hot water. Then comb the oil through the hair with a regular comb. Using a fine toothed comb then comb out the lice and nits. Cover the child's head with a cotton scarf overnight and wash again in the morning. Repeat the treatment if necessary.

- **Echinacea/Goldenseal:** These can be used to improve immune function to prevent infection from occurring.
- **Garlic:** This can help fight the infestation.
- **Tea Tree Oil:** Tea tree oil has strong antiseptic properties and can help rid the scalp of lice. 25 drops of the oil to 1 pint of pure water can be used. Rub in the scalp and comb with a fine-toothed comb to eliminate the lice infestation. The oil can be used three times a day.
- **Blood cleanser formulas** and colon cleansers can help rid the body of toxins on which the parasites feed.

HEADACHE

Headaches can occur at any age and for many different reasons. Rarely is anyone immune from occasional headaches. A young child may not be able to express where the pain is coming from when a headache occurs. A headache can range from mild to extremely painful, as in migraines.

When children complain of headaches, take caution. Watch for recurring headaches, those following an injury, headaches accompanied with fever, any that occur with fainting or loss of consciousness, and those following a convulsion.

CAUSES

Headaches may be caused by a wide range of problems such as muscle tension, an illness, or a disorder with the blood vessels in the head. Some other causes include allergies, illness, fever, high blood pressure, epilepsy, brain tumors, dental problems, drugs or head injury. Headaches that are severe, chronic, cause a stiff neck, leave the child confused, cause fatigue, or accompany a high fever should be taken seriously and medical attention should be sought. This could be a sign of a serious disorder such as meningitis. Some believe that constipation may be a contributing factor to headaches. Make sure the bowels are in good functioning order.

The most common headaches are caused by tension. Tension headaches occur when muscles contract, usually because of emotions. These are usually felt on both sides of the head as well as the back. They are characterized by aching with mild or severe discomfort. They may come on all at once or gradually develop throughout the day. Anxiety, depression, stress, muscle spasms, family problems, or any emotional disturbance can trigger a tension headache.

Vascular headaches are associated with throbbing in the front and sides of the head. These are known as classic migraines and can cause altered vision, sensitivity to light, nausea, and vomiting. They usually recur and cause severe pain. A migraine may last for days and sleep may not even ease the pain. Migraines are associated with different factors including stress, food allergies, hypoglycemia, head injury, hormonal changes or fatigue.

Cluster headaches are known as migrainous cranialneuralgia. This type causes a burning pain which concentrates in the area of the eye with pain traveling to the face or temples.

HOME CARE

- Do not give aspirin to children, as it is associated with the development of Reye's syndrome.
- Have the child relax, lie down in a darkened room, and apply a cool cloth to his head.

- Make sure the child is not constipated as this has been known to cause headaches.
- If the child is under stress, give them extra attention and time to discuss their feelings.

DIETARY GUIDELINES

- Encourage a diet in whole, natural foods.
- Include high fiber foods to protect against constipation.
- Low blood sugar may be a problem, so provide regular, nutritious meals with snacks as needed.
- Avoid foods associated with allergies such as chocolate, dairy, MSG, and other additives.
- Diets high in starches, sugar and meat can cause fermentation in the stomach and toxins to enter the bloodstream, leading to headaches.

NUTRITIONAL SUPPLEMENTS

- **B-Complex:** B-complex vitamins help with stress and emotional problems. A deficiency of vitamin B5 or pantothenic acid may result in headaches and depression.
- **Vitamin E:** It helps supply oxygen to the brain and improves circulation.
- **Acidophilus and Bifidus:** This helps with digestion and can help children who suffer from headaches related to food sensitivities.
- **Calcium and Magnesium:** These are important for muscle relaxation. A deficit has been linked to migraines.

HERBAL REMEDIES

- **Chamomile:** Chamomile tea can help relax the body and relieve muscle tension.
- **Feverfew:** This is helpful when migraines are a problem.
- **Passion Flower:** Passion Flower can help with relaxation and pain.
- **Ginger:** This is known to help in relieving headaches.

HYPERACTIVITY (Attention Deficit Disorder)

Hyperactivity is a condition when the normal exuberance and energy of youth get out of control. It can affect children, adolescence and even some adults. It is characterized by a short attention span, behavioral problems, poor concentration, inappropriate responses, overactivity, and emotional instability.

Some parents feel guilt and responsibility for their child's behavior, but this condition is not a sign of parental failure. It is often embrassing for parents and siblings when the hyperactive child acts inappropriately. This problem can interfere with the life of the entire family. They can easily break and damage things because of overactivity and impulsive behavior as well as injure themselves. These children seem to be in constant motion and are easily frustrated. They may be content and happy one moment and throwing a tantrum the next. One of the most frustrating symptoms is their unpredictable behavior.

The hyperactive child may feel left out by peers. They want to be a part of the group but are often shunned by others. It can be hard for them to fit in with children their age. This may lead them to even more inappropriate behavior by trying to show off.

Approximately two million children have been diagnosed

with hyperactivity. This is about four to twenty percent of the children who are school age. Boys are about four times more often diagnosed with this disorder than girls. These figures are probably not accurate because of the difficulty in diagnosing the condition.

Many parents have found success in treating the hyperactive child with natural foods. Diet changes, natural supplements and herbal remedies have helped the condition in many children.

CAUSES

Hyperactivity is usually thought of as a behavioral disorder of the central nervous system caused by a chemical imbalance in the brain. Most experts believe that there is an insufficient amount of one or more chemicals in the nervous system that are responsible for regulating concentration and attention.

Many natural health practitioners consider hyperactivity to be diet related. It is thought that excessive amounts of sugar can cause chemical imbalances in the body. Sugar has a profound effect on the mind, body and emotions. Children can also react to food additives and pesticides as well. Allergies to milk, wheat, chocolate, yeast, antibiotics and other foods can also cause irrational behavior.

Lead poisoning has been linked to hyperactivity. Lead attacks the brain and nervous system. When inhaled, the lead is assimilated into the blood quickly. Other toxic metals may also cause problems.

Hyperactivity may also be related to vision problems, hearing loss, and communication problems, causing emotional stress. Some children suffering from sleep disorders, lead poisoning, palsy, birth complications, a reaction to medications, prenatal drug abuse, and seizures have been mistakenly diagnosed as being hyperactive.

The hyperactive child is usually of normal or above normal intelligence. But their problems with attention and focusing inhibit them from doing well in school.

HOME CARE

- Have a positive attitude around the hyperactive child. They often feed off of other's emotions.
- Counseling can be beneficial for the entire family, to have everyone become involved and to understand the problem.
- Create a structured, disciplined, routine environment for the child. Be consistent with discipline.
- Be specific when giving the child tasks. Give them one step at a time so they do not feel overwhelmed.
- Exercise may help with hyperactive children. Create positive activities to help use up some of that excess energy.
- Be sure not to neglect other members of the family.

DIETARY GUIDELINES

- Eliminate food additives, refined sugars and artificial sweeteners from the diet. Some hyperactive children may suffer from glucose intolerance. They may also have a tendency toward hypoglycemia. Artificial colors, sweeteners, preservative, stabilizers and all food additives should be eliminated.
- Eliminate foods which may cause allergic reactions.
- Avoid foods that contain salicylates which include almonds, apples, apricots, cherries, currants, berries, peaches, plums, prunes, tomatoes, pickles, green peppers, cucumbers and oranges. Salicylates have been linked to hyperactivity in some children. They are also used as food

additives.

- Studies have shown that hyperactive children on restricted diets show fewer behavior problems in over fifty percent of cases.
- Emphasize vegetables and fruits which do not contain salicylates. Also add whole foods such as oats, rice and millet.

NUTRITIONAL SUPPLEMENTS

- **Calcium and Magnesium:** This combination is soothing and calming on the nervous system. A liquid form can be given to children. Follow the recommended guidelines for different ages.
- **B-Complex Vitamins:** The B-complex vitamins work together in brain function in improving concentration and memory. They also work to calm the nervous system.
- **Vitamin C:** Vitamin C is an anti-stress vitamin and helps strengthen the immune system.
- **Vitamin A:** Vitamin A is strengthening and helps fight allergies.
- **Iron:** Studies have found that an iron deficiency in children can produce symptoms similar to hyperactivity.
- **Multi-Mineral Supplement:** All minerals are needed to protect the brain from the accumulation of heavy metals.
- **GABA:** GABA (gamma-amino butyric acid) has been shown to help in decreasing hyperactivity in children, as well as benefiting children with learning disabilities.
- **Essential Fatty Acids:** The essential fatty acids are important for all body functions and are often lacking in children's diets.
- **Chlorophyll/Blue-Green Algae:** These help to cleanse the blood and provide great nutritional support.

HERBAL REMEDIES

- **Chamomile:** Chamomile tea can help relax the nervous system and calm a child. It may be useful to use before bedtime.
- **Scullcap:** Scullcap is a relaxant and helps in calming the mind and nervous system. It is not recommended for children under the age of six.
- **Valerian:** Valerian can be used in extract form. It is a mild sedative and should be used according to recommended dosages.
- **Gotu Kola:** This is considered a brain food to help with concentration and memory.
- **Hops:** Hops are relaxing and calming on the body.
- **Bee Pollen:** Bee Pollen can help the brain function.
- **Kelp:** Kelp is high in nutritional value and minerals to support brain function.
- **Alfalfa:** This is full of nutrition and aids in eliminating toxins.

IMPETIGO

Impetigo is a contagious condition of the skin caused by streptococcus or staphylococcus bacteria. It can be transmitted from individual to individual by direct contact with the affected area or by touching clothing which has been in contact. Good hygiene is important in avoiding passing the bacteria.

CAUSES

The condition is spread by the fluid from the blisters that form over the affected area. The blisters form a crust that has a yellowish color. When the crust is removed, another one is formed from the fluid underneath. The fluid is what passes impetigo to other individuals. Children are more apt to get the condition. If an infant has impetigo, it should be treated promptly, as it can be very serious and life-threatening to the very young.

Poor hygiene does not cause impetigo as some would believe. Good hygiene is important but it can be spread by coming into direct contact with someone who has the condition.

HOME CARE

- Bathe the child daily to avoid spreading the condition.
- Change sheets, pillow, and towels daily.
- Keep the child from scratching off the crusts, as the fluid under will spread the infection.
- Make sure all children wash hands regularly to avoid spreading or contracting the condition.
- Cut fingernails short to avoid scratching.

DIETARY GUIDELINES

- Avoid refined sugars as they inhibit the body's ability in fighting infection.
- Include nutritious foods such as soups, vegetables, whole grains, and lean meats.

NUTRITIONAL SUPPLEMENTS

- **Acidophilus and Bifidus:** Acidophilus helps reestablish the friendly bacteria into the intestines and helps in the healing process. It should especially be given when a child is on antibiotics.

- **Vitamin C and Bioflavonoids:** These work together in reducing inflammation, stimulating the immune system, and in fighting bacterial infections.
- **Chlorophyll and Blue-Green Algae:** Chlorophyll helps in detoxifying the blood and is rich in essential vitamins and minerals.
- **Zinc:** This can be taken for a few days according to dosage appropriate for different ages.

Herbal Remedies

- **Echinacea:** Echinacea helps stimulate the immune system and fight infections.
- **Golden Seal:** This is a natural antibiotic helpful in healing impetigo. A paste can be put directly on the affected area.
- **Tea Tree Oil:** Tea Tree oil is a strong disinfectant with antibacterial and antifungal properties. A mixture of eight drops of Tea Tree oil with one quart of warm, pure water can be applied to the area.
- **Garlic:** Garlic is healing and has antibacterial properties.
- **Red Clover:** Red Clover helps to purify the blood and eliminate toxins.
- **Kelp:** Kelp contains nutrients for healing.
- **Herbal combinations** for the blood and glands can help.

INFLUENZA

Influenza is caused by a virus that spreads rapidly and affects the upper respiratory tract; sinuses, ears, nose, and throat. The illness is easily spread through coughing and sneezing. It is a viral infection caused by many different viruses. Viruses are capable of changing structure over a period of time, usually two to three years. The flu most commonly occurs during the winter months, often in epidemic proportions.

It usually takes twenty-four to forty-eight hours for the symptoms to appear after exposure. It is highly contagious and symptoms include headache, muscles aches, fatigue, cough, sore throat, lack of appetite, fever, and chills. Diarrhea and an upset stomach may sometimes accompany the flu. The symptoms pass usually in two to three days but may linger for as long as a week.

CAUSES

Influenza is caused by a virus easily spread from person to person. If the immune system is compromised due to stress, lack of sleep, or a poor diet, the body will be more susceptible to infection. It is also a way for the body to rid itself of toxins that build up. Try and make the child as comfortable as possible.

HOME CARE

- Give the child a lot of fluids to help reduce the mucus and prevent dehydration.
- Make the child as comfortable as possible and allow them to rest until they feel better.
- Herbs and natural supplements can help relieve symptoms and speed recovery.

DIETARY GUIDELINES

- Offer fluids, ice chips, or frozen fruit juice to prevent possible dehydration.
- If the child does not want to eat, do not force-feed. A juice fast may help the body heal more rapidly.
- Applesauce, soups, and herbal teas are easy to digest.
- Avoid dairy products, as they can produce excess mucus.
- Warm fluids can help relieve congestion.
- Avoid refined sugars as they can slow the healing process.
- Lemon or lime juice in water can help clear toxins. Add a little honey to taste.

NUTRITIONAL SUPPLEMENTS

- **Vitamin C and Bioflavonoids:** These contain antiviral properties to help heal the infection. There are also anti-inflammatory properties which help reduce the inflammation associated with the flu.
- **Indoles:** Dietary indoles help strengthen the immune system.

HERBAL REMEDIES

- **Chamomile:** Chamomile tea can be given to help the child relax.
- **Echinacea:** Echinacea can help boost the immune system and also contains antiviral properties to heal the infection.
- **Golden Seal:** Golden Seal also contains antiviral properties and aids in healing the mucus membranes.
- **Ginger:** Ginger can help soothe an upset stomach and aids in healing.

- **Garlic:** Garlic is a natural antibiotic which is effective on viral infections. It is also healing and aids in strengthening the immune system.
- **Herbal combinations** for the bowels can help rid the body of toxins.

INSOMNIA

Insomnia in children can be very distressing. A child without enough sleep will be more susceptible to illness, mood changes, depression, may do poorly in school or have dark circles under their eyes. A child may have problems falling asleep or wake during the night, unable to go back to sleep. In either case, it needs to be dealt with. Children do have different sleep requirements, and a very active child may require more sleep. It is important to encourage good sleep habits and watch a child's behavior to make sure they are getting the sleep they need.

Newborns average about sixteen hours of sleep during a twenty-four hour period. School age children require an average of ten to eleven hours of sleep per night. And requirements change as the child grows. Sleep patterns alternate between REM (rapid-eye-movement) and non-REM (a lighter sleep). It is during the REM cycle that dreaming occurs. The cycles vary during a night's sleep, and each cycle is important.

Healthy sleep patterns are important for a growing child. Make bedtime a pleasant time by reading books or having a story time before "lights out." Some people believe that many behavioral problems in children are related to a lack of sleep.

CAUSES

Insomnia in children can be related to many different factors. Growing periods, depression, changes in family, a new house, new friends, anxiety over grades, fear, or many other situations can result in short term insomnia. Stay in touch with each child in order to understand just what they are going through. Talk to them about their fears and problems. Often just relating to a parent who can help them put their concerns in perspective will help in alleviating the problem.

Many believe that nutrition plays a role in this problem. It is also thought that a lack of exercise can lead to insomnia.

HOME CARE

• If a child is having difficulty falling asleep, help them relax and not worry.
• If fear and anxiety are a problem, reassure them and allow the child to discuss their concerns in a loving and caring environment.
• Encourage exercise during the day which can make them more tired in the evening. Avoid exercise at least two hours before bedtime.
• Do not allow a child to eat a heavy meal late in the evening.
• Have the child go to bed at the same time each evening and get up at the same time. Follow a routine as closely as possible.
• Do not give a child sleep medication.
• A fan in a child's room can offer white noise which is soothing and may help them relax and block out other annoying sounds.
• Allow a child to unwind before bedtime. Give him a warm bath and ensure a calm environment.

DIETARY GUIDELINES

- Avoid foods that are stimulating such as caffeine, refined sugar, and chocolate.
- Have dinner early rather than late in the evening.
- A light snack before bedtime may help them to sleep better.
- Foods high in the amino acid tryptophan can help induce sleep. Some include bananas, figs, dates, yogurt, milk, turkey and tuna.

NUTRITIONAL SUPPLEMENTS

- **B-Complex Vitamins:** The B-Complex vitamins help to relax and calm the nervous system.
- **Calcium and Magnesium:** Calcium and Magnesium help to strengthen the nervous system and calm the nerves. A lack of these minerals can lead to insomnia.
- **Vitamin C and Bioflavonoids:** These help to keep the nervous system healthy.

HERBAL REMEDIES

- **Chamomile:** Chamomile tea is mild and can be taken before bedtime to help relax and calm the body.
- **Passion Flower:** This is not recommended for children under four years of age. It is a mild relaxant to promote sleep.
- **Scullcap:** Scullcap can be given as a tea or in extract form to help relax. Avoid with young children.
- **Lobelia:** A small dose of extract can help relax the body.

JAUNDICE

Jaundice is a common condition found in newborn babies. Approximately eighty percent of newborns have some degree of jaundice. This causes a yellowing of the skin, and in the whites of the eyes. In neonatal jaundice of infants, the liver is not yet functioning properly. This is a more common problem in premature babies. It is not usually serious and most often resolves itself within a week.

CAUSES

Jaundice in newborns is caused by a build up of bilirubin in the blood due to a liver that is not yet functioning properly. The red blood cells are fragile in infants. The liver is responsible for converting the cells into bilirubin which then goes to the gall bladder and the bowels. The bilirubin which is not expelled is absorbed into the skin, causing the yellow coloring. It may be a more serious condition when the jaundice involves absence of bile drainage. But this is very rare. Jaundice can be toxic to the brain if the levels are high enough. Slight jaundice is a common problem with newborn babies and is usually of short duration. Rarely there is an incompatibility of blood types between mother and child. The mother's antibodies may destroy the baby's red blood cells.

Jaundice is thought to be more common in children with siblings who had the problem, infants born to diabetics, premature infants, and those with low birth weight.

Home Care

- Expose the baby to sunlight for short periods.
- A health care professional may recommend the baby be placed under artificial bilirubin lights for a period of time.

Dietary Guidelines

- Frequent breast feeding may help to stimulate infant bowel function.
- A nursing mother should eat a high fiber diet.
- A healthy diet for the nursing mother should include fresh fruits and vegetables, whole grains and natural foods.
- Nursing mothers can drink lemon juice and water, beet tops or beet juice.

Nutritional Supplements

- **Multi-Mineral/Vitamin:** This should be taken by the nursing mother to promote health and nutrition.

Herbal Remedies

- **Milk Thistle:** The extract may be beneficial for strengthening the liver. It can be taken by nursing mothers.
- **Dandelion:** This can help build and strengthen the liver when taken by the nursing mother.

183

MEASLES

Measles is a very contagious, viral childhood disease. It usually affects the respiratory system with a fever, runny nose, cough and rash. The rash is splotchy red bumps that may cause extreme itching. It is a typical childhood disease but may also affect adults.

Symptoms occur from ten to fourteen days after exposure. The symptoms usually worsen over a period of a few days. A child with measles is contagious for approximately seven days after symptoms appear. The major concerns center around complications that sometimes follow the measles. These include ear infections, pneumonia, encephalitis, or other infections.

Most children are vaccinated against the measles but there are still a significant number of cases each year among school age children.

CAUSES

Measles are passed by coughing or sneezing, with droplets from the throat or mouth coming into contact with another individual. It can also be contracted by touching bedding, towels, or articles of clothing from an infected person. It is an acute disease and may be a natural means in the body of getting rid of toxins. Natural remedies can help ease the symptoms as the condition runs its course.

HOME CARE

- Encourage fluids, especially when a fever is present, to protect against dehydration.
- Keep the lights dim as the child's eyes may be sensitive.
- Watch for signs of secondary infection.

- Make the child as comfortable as possible.
- Apply creams to help soothe the itching.
- Keep young children's fingernails short to avoid scarring from itching.
- A cornstarch bath may help soothe the itching.

Dietary Guidelines

- Juices should be encouraged. A sore throat may be soothed by fruit juice popsicles, fruit juices, herbal teas, or soups.
- Eliminate refined sugars as they slow the healing process.
- Eliminate fats which are hard for the body to digest.
- Stick to fluids if they do not want solid food for a few days.
- Pure water should be used.

Nutritional Supplements

- **Calcium and Magnesium:** Calcium and Magnesium help to promote tissue healing and can be relaxing and calming.
- **Vitamin A:** Vitamin A helps with healing, boosting the immune system and in healing the mucous membranes.
- **Vitamin C and Bioflavonoids:** These work together to reduce inflammation and stimulate the immune function.
- **Zinc:** Zinc can help stimulate the immune system but should be used as directed and for a short period of time.
- **Vitamin E:** Vitamin E helps boost the immune system and heal the skin.

HERBAL REMEDIES

- **Echinacea:** Echinacea can help strengthen the immune system and has antiviral properties.
- **Chamomile:** Chamomile tea can help reduce fever and relax the body.
- **Catnip:** Catnip tea helps to relax the body.
- **Herbal laxatives** can be given if constipation develops.

MOTION SICKNESS

Motion sickness is fairly common in children when traveling either by car, boat, plane or train. It can interrupt a vacation or spoil a short trip to the store. It is characterized by mild to severe nausea, sometimes causing vomiting. The child may become uneasy, pale, quiet, dizzy, or complain of a headache. Once motion sickness occurs, it usually takes a few hours for the child to fully recover.

Prevention is important with motion sickness. Avoid junk foods, alcohol and heavy foods before traveling. Avoid strong food odors and smoke. Keep the air cool if possible.

CAUSES

Motion sickness is caused by an overstimulation of the vestibular apparatus of the inner ear which is responsible for maintaining balance. Some children are more sensitive to this condition. The eyes and inner ear contribute to a sense of balance. An imbalance is created when these two systems send different messages to the brain. Nausea can occur when the brain cannot figure out what to do. It may be a sign that the digestive system is in a weakened condition. There may be accumulations of toxins or mucus, causing an imbalance in the system.

Home Care

- Use whatever treatment works for the child before leaving home.
- Take remedies in the car.
- Fresh air circulating in the car may help prevent motion sickness.
- Sitting in the front seat helps some children.
- Don't allow a susceptible child to read or play games while traveling in a moving vehicle.
- Try and keep the child calm and distracted while the vehicle is in motion.

Dietary Guidelines

- Avoid dairy products which cause mucus.
- Avoid fatty foods that may upset the stomach.
- Some children do better on a full stomach and others on an empty stomach, so watch your child and prepare accordingly.

Nutritional Supplements

- **Acidophilus and Bifidus:** This helps in the digestion of food.
- **Vitamin A:** Vitamin A is healing and helps strengthen the mucous membranes.
- **B-Complex Vitamins:** These help relax the body and may help when a child is feeling stress.

HERBAL REMEDIES

- **Ginger:** Ginger is very effective for motion sickness. Studies have confirmed its value even above that of over-the-counter medications. It can be taken in capsule form or as a tea for younger children. It should be taken first one half hour before leaving and then can be given every two hours while traveling.
- **Hops:** This is a natural sedative that works to calm and relax the stomach.
- **Red Raspberry:** Red Raspberry is useful for conditions such as nausea and vomiting.
- **St. John's Wort:** It helps to relax a nervous stomach.
- **Herbal combinations** for the liver, blood and colon may help clear toxins from the system if necessary.

MUMPS

Mumps is a viral infection which causes swelling in the parotids which are two of the salivary glands located below the ears. It is most commonly found in children between the ages of four to fifteen but can occur in older individuals. It can cause serious complications in young men as it can attack the testicles and in some cases cause sterility. Mumps is rarely seen in children because of the vaccination most receive. Infection can occur before the onset of the symptoms until after the glands return to normal size. Immunity occurs from infection. After exposure through contact with infectious saliva, symptoms occur from two to three and a half weeks.

A high fever, fatigue and headache usually precede the swelling. Within two days the jaw may become stiff and painful and swelling occurs in the parotid glands. The swelling most often lasts from three to seven days. In some cases one gland may swell first and the other swell ten to twelve days later.

Causes

Mumps is caused by a viral infection affecting the parotid glands. Swelling occurs in one or both of the parotid glands at the jaws.

Home Care

- Try and make the child as comfortable as possible.
- Apply cool or warm compresses to the swollen area to ease the pain.
- Young men should rest as much as possible to avoid testicular problems.
- Isolate the child as much as possible to avoid spreading the infection to others.
- Watch for signs of a secondary infection.
- Perspiration can help eliminate toxins through the skin.

Dietary Guidelines

- Soft foods are easier to eat when there is swelling and pain. Applesauce and yogurt are easy to digest.
- Fluids should be given such as pure water, citrus juices, herbal teas, vegetable broths and soups. Fruit juice popsicles can feel good on the throat.
- Fats should be avoided as they are hard to digest.
- Avoid refined sugars as they slow the healing process.

Nutritional Supplements

- **Vitamin A and Beta-Carotene:** These help in healing the mucous membranes and in building the immune system.

- **Vitamin C and Bioflavonoids:** These help strengthen the immune system and help the healing process. They help to destroy the virus.
- **Acidophilus and Bifidus:** This helps with the digestion process and in encouraging the growth of beneficial bacteria.
- **Indoles:** Dietary indoles help strengthen the immune system.

HERBAL REMEDIES

- **Chamomile:** Chamomile tea can help the child relax when they are uncomfortable.
- **Mullein:** Mullein is a traditional remedy used for viral infections.
- **Echinacea:** Echinacea contains anti-viral properties and will strengthen the immune system to aid in the healing process.
- **Red Clover:** A tea can be sweetened with a little honey and helps in cleaning the blood.
- **Lobelia:** Lobelia can help relax the body and loosen mucus if it is a problem.
- **Myrrh:** Myrrh contains antiseptic properties to help with healing.
- **Herbal combinations** for the colon and kidneys may help eliminate toxins.

NAUSEA AND VOMITING

Nausea occurs often in babies and young children. It is usually a symptom rather than an actual illness. It may begin with cramps or pain, a loss of appetite, or fatigue. Vomiting or diarrhea may occur after the initial pain.

CAUSES

Nausea and vomiting can be caused by many physical and emotional problems. Infants may vomit with any imbalance in their systems such as an infection. It may be the sign of a serious problem and should be watched carefully. Older children may get nauseated and vomit for a variety of reasons such as motion sickness, eating rich foods, overeating, food poisoning, fatigue, constipation, infection, appendicitis, food allergies, nervousness, homesickness, or anger. Vomiting is one means that the body has of eliminating toxins and mucus from the stomach. Emotional problems can often be a reason for nausea. A new sibling, tension in the home, divorce, and even anticipation of an upcoming trip or holiday can cause nausea.

HOME CARE

• If the problem seems to be emotional in nature, allow the child to talk and discuss their concerns either with a parent, mature adult friend, therapist, school counselor, or religious leader.
• Be aware of the possibility of dehydration, especially in babies, and offer clear fluids.
• A hot water bottle may help relieve stomach discomfort.

DIETARY GUIDELINES

• Fluids should be given to avoid dehydration. Infants and young children can become dehydrated easily with vomiting and diarrhea. Sipping fluids or sucking on ice chips or a fruit popsicle can help. Pure water, fruit juice or herbal teas can be given.

- Clear liquids can be given when vomiting occurs to replace some of the lost fluid.
- The child will ask for food when they are ready. Soft, bland foods should be offered first such as applesauce, yogurt, dry toast, or soup.
- Brown Rice water is nutritious and healing.

NUTRITIONAL SUPPLEMENTS

- **Acidophilus and Bifidus:** This helps to encourage the growth of beneficial bacteria in the intestinal tract and aids in digestion.
- **Chlorophyll/Blue-Green Algae:** These can help cleanse the stomach and nourish the body.

HERBAL REMEDIES

- **Peppermint:** Peppermint tea is calming on the stomach.
- **Ginger:** Ginger in capsule or tea form is soothing on the stomach and helps relieve nausea.
- **Aloe Vera:** Aloe Vera juice can help a sour stomach.
- **Chamomile:** Chamomile tea helps relax the child and soothe the stomach.
- **Alfalfa:** Alfalfa will provide nourishment, and calm and strengthen the stomach.
- **An herbal extract formula** containing Scullcap, Passion Flower, Wild Yam, Valerian, Myrrh Gum or other relaxants, help to calm the nerves.

NOSEBLEEDS

Nosebleeds commonly occur in children and are usually not serious. The blood vessels in the front part of the nose are close to the surface and can easily be damaged and burst. Blood loss is usually minimal though it may look like a lot. Keep the child in a sitting position or with head raised. Hold tissue under the nostrils. The nose can be pinched for a few minutes. The child may be frightened by the sight of blood so reassure and comfort them. Healing will occur quickly, usually within a week.

CAUSES

A nosebleed can be caused by an injury to the nose. A fall off a bike or fight with a friend can cause the problem. It can be painful. Allergies can cause swelling in the nasal passages, making them more susceptible to bleeding. Some children even wake up with blood on their pillow, sheets and clothing. A lack of humidity may cause the nasal membranes to crack and bleed. Children with serious medical conditions such as high blood pressure, hemophilia and leukemia may be more susceptible, so ask a medical professional for advice.

HOME CARE

- Have the child sit up or lie down with the head raised.
- Tilt the head forward.
- Have the child breathe through their mouth.
- Apply pressure with a finger and thumb to the bridge of the nose, allowing a clot to form. Do this for five to ten minutes and check to see if the bleeding has stopped.
- If bleeding continues after thirty minutes, seek medical assistance.

- An icepack can be applied to the bridge of the nose to constrict the blood vessels and control the bleeding.
- Tissue can be placed under the nose to catch the blood.
- Reassure the child. They may be frightened by the sight of the blood.
- Use a humidifier if the air is dry.
- One teaspoon of vinegar in a cup of pure water can help stop a nosebleed.

DIETARY GUIDELINES

- After the bleeding stops, fluids can be given.

NUTRITIONAL SUPPLEMENTS

- **Vitamin K:** Vitamin K is known as the clotting vitamin. It is found in green leafy vegetables such as kale and spinach.
- **Vitamin C and Bioflavonoids:** Vitamin C with Bioflavonoids help strengthen the capillaries and aid healing.
- **B-Complex Vitamins:** These will help with healing.
- **Chlorophyll/Blue-Green Algae:** These contain vitamin K to help with clotting.

HERBAL REMEDIES

- **Aloe Vera:** Aloe Vera gel can be placed in the nose to relieve dryness.
- **Horsetail:** This helps promote blood coagulation. Avoid giving to small children.

OBESITY

The number of overweight children continues to increase. Obesity is defined as weighing twenty percent over the average for age, sex and size. Obesity as a child can lead to obesity as an adult. This results in a greater risk of many diseases such as heart disease and diabetes. Obesity is a complex problem and involves more than just eating too much. Other factors include; lack of exercise, genetics, cultural background, physical characteristics, and social or economic status.

CAUSES

The most common causes of obesity center around a lack of exercise combined with overeating. A diet high in refined carbohydrates and fat but low in fiber can lead to obesity. Children left home alone look to convenience foods which are often not healthy. They also watch television and play video games, rather than doing activities which allow for movement and use of energy.

Genetics seem to predispose some individuals to obesity. But this may be due to learned eating patterns as well as genetics. It is certainly important for children to see their parents exercising and eating healthy foods. Teaching children healthy lifestyle patterns will aid them in achieving proper weight patterns.

HOME CARE

• Do not make the child feel self conscious about their weight. This can lead to serious problems such as anorexia and bulimia.

- Have healthy, nutritious foods on hand for the child to eat.
- Watch for signs of depression that may be associated with overeating.
- Look for other emotional problems in children. They may be seeking comfort through eating.
- Exercise should be enjoyable for a child. Participate with them in activities such as walking, biking, basketball, or any activity. Teenagers may want to join a local health club.
- Encourage children to talk about their feelings and emotions.
- Avoid chewing gum, as it activates the gastric juices and produces feelings of hunger.
- Encourage a calm environment when eating. Chew food slowly and thoroughly.
- Permanent weight loss takes time, so be positive and supportive to the child if they are trying to lose weight.

DIETARY GUIDELINES

- Encourage the child to drink six to eight glasses of pure water a day. This can help avoid constipation and flush toxins from the body.
- Tell the child to eat when they feel hungry.
- Avoid fad diets and encourage a slow, permanent approach to weight loss.
- Children need healthy foods. Offer fresh fruits and vegetables, whole grains, lean meats, and fiber rich foods.
- Avoid refined sugar products, chocolate, soda, caffeine, and additives in food.
- Cook low fat, healthy meals for the entire family.

NUTRITIONAL SUPPLEMENTS

- **Multi-Vitamin/Mineral:** Give the child a vitamin/mineral supplement.
- **Chromium:** This helps to regulate blood sugar levels. It has also been found to help reduce cravings for sweets.
- **B-Complex Vitamins:** The B-complex vitamins help with appetite regulation.
- **Essential Fatty Acids:** The essential fatty acids have been known to help with weight loss. They are important for overall health in children, as well.
- **L-methionine, Choline, Inositol:** These amino acids help with appetite suppression, blood sugar levels, and fat metabolism.

HERBAL REMEDIES

- **Licorice:** Licorice root can help reduce cravings for sweets and strengthen the adrenal glands. Licorice should not be given to children with high blood pressure because of possible complications.
- **Red Raspberry:** Red Raspberry tea may help reduce the appetite and increase energy.
- **Dandelion:** Dandelion root is considered a liver tonic. Liver function may have some effect on weight. Dandelion has been used successfully to promote weight loss.
- **Red Clover:** Red Clover can help clear toxins from the body that may contribute to excess weight.
- **Ginseng:** Ginseng aids in controlling blood sugar levels, increasing energy and in reducing cravings for sweets.
- **An herbal combination** for the colon can help prevent intestinal congestion.

PARASITES AND WORMS

Parasites and worms are common in children. Youngsters from ages two to six spend a lot of time exploring the outside world, often putting their hands in the mouth. Parasites can be found both inside and outside the body. They are most commonly found in hot, humid climates. Infestation occurs as the eggs settle in the intestines and enter the body. They can also be passed to children through pets. There are over three hundred different types of parasites in the United States. Some include tapeworms, pinworms, hookworms, whipworms, roundworms and Giardia lamblia.

CAUSES

If the child is weak or has a poor digestive system, infestation is more likely. When the digestive system is in good condition, the hydrochloric acid will destroy the parasites and worms. Ingestion of larvae or eggs from partially cooked meat, especially pork, can cause the problem. Walking barefoot through the dirt or ingesting soil can cause infestation. Giardia lamblia, a microscopic organism, has been found in some drinking water. It is also found in streams that have been frequented by animals. Raw meat, especially pork, may contain parasites. So use good sanitary measures when handling raw meat and cook properly. Antibiotics and immune-suppressing drugs reduce the beneficial bacteria in the intestines and may allow an environment for parasites and worms. Pinworms are one of the most common parasites. Its eggs are usually ingested and transferred by fingernails, clothing, bedding and food.

HOME CARE

- Have the child wash their hands after playing outside or touching animals.
- Keep the fingernails short and clean.
- Check the child's stool if infestation is suspected.
- When cooking and handling raw meat, use Clorox to wash hands and clean surfaces.

DIETARY GUIDELINES

- Fresh carrot juice, given one hour before meals, can help.
- Add garlic to food. It can help kill the parasites.
- Avoid refined sugar and its products. The parasites will thrive on sugar products.
- Encourage a diet of green leafy vegetables, vegetables and fruits, whole grains, and nutritious foods.
- Pumpkin seeds can help destroy the invaders.
- Encourage a high fiber diet which can help cleanse the colon.

NUTRITIONAL SUPPLEMENTS

- **Vitamin C and Bioflavonoids:** Vitamin C and Bioflavonoids help build the immune system and heal.
- **B-Complex Vitamins:** The B-Complex vitamins help digestion and in detoxifying the liver.
- **Iodine:** This is found in kelp and helps kill parasites and worms.
- **Acidophilus and Bifidus:** Acidophilus helps provide beneficial bacteria which may be affected by parasites in the intestines.
- **Chlorophyll/Blue-Green Algae:** This helps with digestion and in cleansing the blood.

HERBAL REMEDIES

- **Cascara Sagrada:** Cascara Sagrada helps with waste elimination.
- **Garlic:** Garlic helps expel worms and parasites. It is antiparasitic.
- **Black Walnut:** Black Walnut is known for its ability to kill parasites in the digestive tract. An extract can be used but should be avoided by infants and small children.
- **Wormwood:** This helps in killing parasites in the intestines.
- **Horsetail:** Horsetail helps kill parasites and worm eggs.
- **Echinacea/Golden Seal:** These help destroy worms and parasites.
- **Herbal combinations** for the colon and parasites can help with the problem.

PNEUMONIA

Pneumonia used to be one of the most dreaded diseases known. Though it is still a serious illness, it is rarely fatal except in those with severely weakened immune systems. It involves inflammation and infection of the lung tissue, resulting in fluid filling the tiny air sacs.

Pneumonia usually begins with a respiratory infection from a flu or cold. It can progress quickly or gradually. It generally causes a fever, headache, malaise, chills, cough, rapid breathing, nausea, vomiting, sweating and chest pain. The cough is usually not productive until the later stages of the disease. There may be a bluish tinge to the skin. A viral infection may progress to a bacterial infection if it is left untreated.

Bacterial pneumonia comes on suddenly often following

another illness. It can be very serious. The child will feel sick, have a high fever, difficulty in breathing, chills, pain, and a cough. Recovery may take two to three weeks. And a cough and fatigue may continue for up to two months.

CAUSES

Pneumonia can be caused by a bacteria, virus, fungi, or mycoplasma. They enter the lungs and cause inflammation. When the epiglottis, which protects the lungs, becomes weakened, as in cases of surgery, loss of consciousness, or seizure, microbes can invade the lungs increasing the risk of infection. A weakened immune system can increase the risk of pneumonia. Other factors include exposure to smoke, asthma, malnutrition, kidney failure, and respiratory infections. It is a common secondary infection with influenza and AIDS.

Viruses known to cause pneumonia are Adenovirus, the Syncytial virus and Coxsackievirus. Bacterial pneumonia is often caused by Pneumococci, Staphylococci and Chlamydia.

If the kidneys and colon are weak, toxins will be eliminated through the lungs causing irritations. Air pollution can cause respiratory illnesses such as asthma, allergies, bronchitis and pneumonia. It can also cause scarring in the lungs which can leave an individual more susceptible to conditions such as pneumonia.

HOME CARE

- A child with pneumonia needs extra fluid intake. This will thin the mucus secretions and encourage a productive cough.
- Increase moisture by using a cool air humidifier.
- Do not suppress the cough as it helps bring up the mucus.
- A hot water bottle on the chest can help relieve pain.
- Rest is necessary to aid in recovery.

DIETARY GUIDELINES

- Offer the child large amounts of pure water, diluted fruit juice, vegetable juice, soup, and herbal tea.
- Avoid refined sugar, fatty foods, and caffeine.
- Avoid dairy products which can increase the production of mucus.
- Encourage the child to eat natural foods when ready to eat. It won't hurt them to take only liquids for a few days. This can help cleanse the body. The child will usually ask for food when they are ready.

NUTRITIONAL SUPPLEMENTS

- **Vitamin C and Bioflavonoids:** These are healing and can help the immune system in fighting the infection. They should be taken at the onset of the illness. Vitamin C has anti-inflammatory properties.
- **Vitamin A/Beta-Carotene:** These help boost the immune system, soothe the mucous membranes, and promote healing.
- **Acidophilus and Bifidus:** This is especially important to restore beneficial bacteria if undergoing antibiotic therapy.
- **Vitamin E:** Vitamin E helps to heal and protect the lungs.
- **Zinc:** Zinc can be given for up to two weeks following directions. It help immune function and tissue repair.

HERBAL REMEDIES

- **Comfrey/Fenugreek:** These help in combination to break up the mucus in the lungs.
- **Ginger:** A tea can be made to help break up the mucus, increase circulation and relieve the fever.
- **Garlic:** Garlic contains antibiotic properties and helps

with the healing process.
- **Marshmallow:** Marshmallow is soothing to the lungs.
- **Mullein:** Mullein helps improve the circulation of the lymphatic system.
- **Thyme:** Thyme is good for lung infections to clear mucus.
- **Echinacea:** This has antibiotic properties and helps immune function.

POISON IVY/POISON OAK

The allergic reaction caused by exposure to plants such as poison ivy and poison oak can be extremely annoying and severe in some individuals. The rash occurs after the skin comes in contact with the resin contained in the leaves, stem and roots of the plant. This oily substance is a potent natural toxin. It only takes a small amount of resin to cause a serious reaction.

Poison ivy and oak can be contracted through touching a person, object or animal that has made contact with the plant. Some highly susceptible individuals can even contract the rash from smoke of burning plants. If the leaves are eaten, a serious mouth poisoning can result. The most common parts of the body affected are the hands, legs, arms, and face. It is not spread by scratching the blisters. The oil of the plant must be present to spread the rash.

A child may come into contact with the plant after playing in the woods, or in some parts of the country, just in their backyards. It can even be found in the grass and mowed with the lawn. The rash may appear from two hours to two days after exposure. The rash usually lasts from one to four weeks. The severity of the reaction will depend on the sensitivity of the child as well as the exposure time. If a child comes in contact with the plant, it is important to wash the child with soap and water and the clothing they were wearing in hot water.

The rash develops first as red, small pimples that itch and develop into a blister filled with fluid. In some cases, the blisters will begin to weep. Itching and burning usually occur and can cause severe discomfort. Though the affected area looks awful, it rarely results in scarring. Keep the area clean to avoid possible infection. If a serious reaction occurs, seek medical attention.

CAUSES

The oil sap contained in the bark, roots, leaves and stem of the plants cause the allergic reaction to the human skin. Some children seem to be immune to the reaction while some suffer serious problems from exposure. This oil is considered one of the most powerful toxins requiring only a small amount to cause a reaction.

HOME CARE

- If exposure is suspected, wash the child carefully as soon as possible with soap and water. Wash all clothing as well. Alcohol can also be rubbed on the area.
- Very hot showers can help remove the histamines, allowing the itching to be relieved for a few hours. This will be helpful before bedtime.
- Calamine lotion can help relieve itching.
- Ice packs or frozen vegetable bags can be placed on the rash to relieve itching and inflammation.
- A baking soda and water paste can be placed on the affected area.
- Cucumber slices can be applied to the area to relieve itching and promote healing.

Dietary Guidelines

- Fluids such as pure water, diluted fruit juice and herbal teas will help flush the system of toxins.
- Avoid sugar products that can slow healing.
- Encourage a healthy diet full of fruits and vegetables.

Nutritional Supplements

- **Vitamin C and Bioflavonoids:** These help the immune system in healing and fighting infection. It can also help with the itching and inflammation.
- **Vitamin A/Beta-Carotene:** These help heal, build new tissue and boost the immune system.
- **Vitamin E:** Used both internally and externally can help promote healing of the skin tissue.
- **Chlorophyll/Blue-Green Algae:** These will help nourish the body and clean the liver, kidneys, blood and colon.
- **Calcium and Magnesium:** A deficiency may make a child more susceptible to skin irritations.

Herbal Remedies

- **Aloe Vera:** The gel can be applied to heal and relieve itching and pain.
- **Jewelweed:** Jewelweed juice can be applied to the area to relieve itching and inflammation.
- **Milkweed:** Juice from the Milkweed can be applied to the area to aid in controlling itching.
- **Echinacea:** This can help prevent infection and build immunity when taken internally.
- **Garlic:** Garlic can help prevent infection and promote healing.

PRECOCIOUS PUBERTY

Precocious puberty is a condition found mainly in females where the onset of puberty is unusually early. Changes such as breast development, pubic hair and menstruation may begin before age nine. The average age is thirteen. Males may begin to mature sexually around the age of ten years.

CAUSES

Precocious puberty has been linked to various factors, one of which is the use of hormones in animals. These excess hormones are ingested by children from chicken, beef, pork and dairy products. Other contributing factors may include tumors, infection, and trauma.

HOME CARE

• Encourage a healthy diet.
• Avoid drugs as much as possible.
• Encourage exercise as it can help with the metabolism of fat and aid in normalizing hormone balance.

DIETARY GUIDELINES

• Avoid meat that has been treated with hormones.
• Encourage a diet full of fruits, vegetables, and natural foods.
• Avoid fatty foods.
• Fresh salads, cabbage, garlic, onions, parsley, carrots and broccoli are beneficial for health.

NUTRITIONAL SUPPLEMENTS

- **Vitamin A:** This can help heal and strengthen the mucous membranes.
- **Vitamin E:** Vitamin E is known to help with hormone imbalance.
- **Vitamin C and Bioflavonoids:** These help to increase healing and cleanse the body.
- **B-Complex:** These vitamins are needed on a daily basis to help the body deal with stress and for healing.

HERBAL REMEDIES

- **Dong Quai:** This helps to balance the hormones.
- **Kelp:** Kelp is high in many nutrients to help the body. It also helps to balance hormones and contains natural iodine.
- **Licorice:** This helps with hormone balance. It should be used with caution in children with low blood sugar.

PSORIASIS

Psoriasis is a skin condition in which the skin cell production gets out of control. It is commonly seen as thickened patches of inflamed skin. The condition can affect large sections of the skin, causing embarrassment and discomfort for children. The tendency toward psoriasis is thought to be hereditary. The symptoms usually appear slowly during childhood. The condition affects different individuals in different ways. It is less common during the summer months. It is not contagious.

CAUSES

Psoriasis is hereditary in some cases, though there is no exact known cause. Attacks have been linked to emotional stress, food allergies, surgery, physical illness, immune disorders, liver problems, or a trauma to the skin. If the kidneys and colon are congested, this may contribute to skin disorders.

There are three main types of psoriasis which include:

Discoid or plaque psoriasis:
This type is characterized by thick, scaly patches on the trunk and limbs. The elbows, knees and scalp are often affected.

Guttate psoriasis:
This occurs most often in children. It consists of red patches of inflamed skin that develop quickly and spread.

Pustular psoriasis:
This consists of small pustules that appear anywhere on the body or just in the palms of the hands or bottoms of the feet.

HOME CARE

- Keep the skin moisturized. Cream can be applied to the area and covered with plastic overnight.
- Exposure to sunlight may be beneficial. Avoid getting burned.
- Oatmeal based soaps can be useful because they do not dry out the skin.
- Avoid stress as much as possible. Encourage children to talk about their concerns.
- Skin brushing may help encourage elimination of toxins.

- Wash the skin with a clean cloth each time to avoid bacterial growth on the cloth.

DIETARY GUIDELINES

- Avoid foods which commonly cause food allergies such as dairy and wheat products.
- Eliminate sugar and other refined foods.
- Encourage a diet which is nutritionally sound such as fruits, vegetables, and whole grains. Avoid wheat if sensitive.
- Juice fasting for a few days may help clean the body of toxins.

NUTRITIONAL SUPPLEMENTS

- **Flaxseed Oil:** This can be applied directly to the affected area to promote healing.
- **Ginger:** Ginger can be added to a warm bath with a few teaspoons of olive oil to soothe and heal.
- **Vitamin A:** This helps promote healing and healthy skin.
- **Vitamin D:** This aids in healing the skin.
- **Vitamin C:** Vitamin C participates in the formation of connective tissue and collagen.
- **B-Complex Vitamins:** The B-Complex vitamins help the body deal with stress as well as aid in maintaining healthy skin.

HERBAL REMEDIES

- **Lavender:** This can be combined with olive oil and applied to the affected areas.

- **Dandelion:** Dandelion helps detoxify the liver which needs to be healthy to avoid chronic skin conditions.
- **Golden Seal:** Golden Seal inhibits the formation of polyamines that result from digestive problems and may be linked to psoriasis.
- **Red Clover:** This helps purify the blood of toxins. A wet compress can be applied externally to control inflammation.
- **Herbal combinations** can help such as kidney and colon formulas.

RASHES

Rashes can appear from time to time for no apparent reason. Skin irritations are rarely life threatening. The skin is a protection for the child from heat, cold and the environment. It also is a method of eliminating toxins from the body.

CAUSES

Rashes can occur from a variety of causes. Heat, food allergies, stress, plants, food additives, metals, chemicals, and just about anything may induce an allergic reaction which develops into a rash. Remove the allergen if it is known. Many natural health professionals consider rashes to be caused by poisons in the body attempting to be eliminated through the skin. If the condition persists without a known cause, it may be wise to consult a medical practitioner.

HOME CARE

- Keep the area clean to protect against infection.
- Oatmeal based soaps can help soothe and moisten the skin.
- Check the child's diet to see if any new foods have been introduced.
- Watch the child to see if they are getting enough sleep, have energy, and if any other symptoms accompany the rash.

DIETARY GUIDELINES

- Eliminate common allergy producing foods such as dairy, wheat, chocolate, preservatives, additives, food colorings and fatty foods.
- Encourage high fluid intake to help clear toxins from the body. Pure water and diluted fruit juices can be given.
- Serve natural, whole foods to the child.

NUTRITIONAL SUPPLEMENTS

- **Vitamin A:** Vitamin A helps heal the skin and strengthen the immune system.
- **Acidophilus and Bifidus:** Acidophilus helps with digestion and in increasing the beneficial bacteria in the digestive tract.
- **Vitamin D:** This helps in healing the skin.
- **Vitamin C:** Vitamin C helps in strengthening the immune system and in healing.

HERBAL REMEDIES

- **Burdock:** Burdock can help clear toxins and is useful in healing rashes.
- **Red Clover:** This helps in clearing the blood of toxins.
- **Calendula:** Calendula is a great healing agent for rashes.
- **Chickweed:** Chickweed has anti-inflammatory and healing properties.
- **Echinacea:** Echinacea helps in healing and improving the immune system.

REYE'S SYNDROME

Reye's Syndrome has been associated with the use of aspirin during common childhood diseases. The exact cause is not known but may occur after a viral illness. Studies seem to indicate that 95 percent of children who get Reye's Syndrome were given aspirin during a viral illness. It was also noted that the more aspirin taken, the more severe the condition. It is a relatively rare disorder but very serious in nature. It usually occurs in children under the age of eighteen following an illness. It is an extremely serious condition, even life threatening, that involves vital body organs, most often the brain and liver but in rarer instances the pancreas, heart, kidneys, spleen and lymph nodes.

The symptoms of the illness will appear as the child is recovering from a virus, usually two days to two weeks after. Symptoms include vomiting, fever, lethargy, fatigue, headache, paralysis, speech impairment, vision problems, delirium, confusion, seizures, heart problems, coma, breathing difficulties, and jaundice. The disease progresses rapidly into a serious condition.

CAUSES

The cause of Reye's Syndrome is unknown, but in 95 percent of the cases the children were given aspirin during treatment for a viral illness.

HOME CARE

- Avoid giving aspirin to children under the age of twenty one.
- Get medical care immediately as it is a life threatening condition.

DIETARY GUIDELINES

- After emergency treatment has been given and the child is recovering, gradually introduce natural, whole foods.
- Avoid refined sugar, additives, and preservatives.

NUTRITIONAL SUPPLEMENTS

- Wait until the child is home from the hospital before gradually introducing immune-building supplements.

HERBAL REMEDIES

- After the child is home from the hospital, herbal remedies can be used to aid in healing and recovery.

RHEUMATIC FEVER

Rheumatic fever occurs as a complication from a strep infection or scarlet fever. It is most commonly seen in children between the ages of four and eighteen. It is characterized by a fever, pain, swelling and redness in the joints, a rash on the trunk and limbs, twitching of the limbs, and bumps on the joints, spine or scalp. The most serious reason for concern centers around the possibility of carditis, an inflammation of the heart tissue which can cause permanent heart damage to the valves.

The symptoms usually appear anywhere from seven to twenty-eight days after strep throat. And the recovery process may take as long as three months. Once a child has had rheumatic fever they should be treated promptly if strep is ever suspected.

CAUSES

Rheumatic fever occurs as a complication of a streptococcus infection as in cases of strep throat, tonsillitis or scarlet fever. When toxins accumulate in the body, it is easier for infections to occur. Many children carry strep bacteria in their throats but they don't usually have problems unless the immune system is inhibited.

HOME CARE

- If your child has strep, watch for any complications.
- Seek medical attention immediately to prevent any permanent heart damage.
- Rest is essential in the healing process.
- Follow instructions from a health care professional.

214

Dietary Guidelines

- Fluid intake should be increased. This helps in flushing toxins from the body. Pure water, warm soup, diluted juices, and herbal teas may be given.
- Citrus juices are healing.
- Eliminate mucus forming foods.
- Avoid refined sugars and products as well as dairy while the child is recovering.
- Encourage a natural diet full of fresh fruits and vegetables as well as whole grains.

Nutritional Supplements

- **Vitamin C and Bioflavonoids:** These help strengthen the immune system, reduce inflammation, protect the mucous membranes and aid in the healing process.
- **Vitamin A/Beta-Carotene:** These aid the immune function as well as the healing process.
- **Calcium and Magnesium:** This combination can help with joint pain from the rheumatic fever.
- **Vitamin E:** This can help protect the heart from scar tissue and damage.
- **Potassium:** Potassium will help protect the heart from damage.
- **Zinc:** This can help with healing and in preventing scarring. It should be given for short periods of time following instructions on the label.
- **Chlorophyll/Blue-Green Algae:** These can help purify the blood and remove toxins from the body.
- **Indoles:** Dietary indoles can help strengthen the immune system.

HERBAL REMEDIES

- **Red Clover:** This can help rid the blood of toxins.
- **Garlic:** Garlic contains antibacterial properties to help with the infection.
- **Echinacea:** Echinacea can help with the healing process and contains antibacterial properties.
- **Chamomile:** Chamomile tea can help relax the child to aid in resting and healing.
- **Catnip:** This can also help the child relax.
- **Comfrey and Fenugreek:** These help in eliminating mucus buildup in the body.
- **Herbal laxative combinations** and blood purifiers can help.

RINGWORM

Ringworm is a fungal infection of the outer layers of the skin. It is highly contagious and is passed easily between classmates and neighborhoods. It can also be spread by stray animals. Ringworm is usually in a ring shape on the skin and is scaly and red. It can spread from one part of the body to another. It is not a serious condition but should be treated.

CAUSES

Ringworm is caused by a fungus spread via other individuals, animals, bedding, shower stalls, etc. It is the same fungus that causes athlete's foot.

Home Care

- The child's skin should be kept clean and dry as fungus prefers a warm, moist environment.
- Clean bedding, towels, clothing, and shower stalls daily to prevent spreading of the fungus.

Dietary Guidelines

- Avoid refined sugars and products.
- Encourage natural foods such as fruits, vegetables and whole grains to make the body as healthy, and less desirable to the fungus, as possible.
- Vegetables are especially good because of their high content of minerals and vitamins.

Nutritional Supplements

- **Vitamin C and Bioflavonoids:** These will help speed healing and strengthen the immune system.
- **Vitamin E:** This is healing and soothing on the skin. It can be taken internally or applied to the affected area.
- **Vitamin A/Beta-Carotene:** These will help speed the healing.

Herbal Remedies

- **Tea Tree Oil:** Tea Tree oil contains antifungal properties and has been shown to be effective in fighting ringworm. Eight drops of the oil should be combined with one pint of pure water and then applied to the area three times daily.
- **Echinacea:** This can help the immune system in fighting the fungus.

- **Red Clover:** Red Clover is useful in eliminating toxins from the blood.
- **Black Walnut:** This can help by applying the extract to the ringworm.
- **Golden Seal:** Golden Seal contains antibiotic properties and can be used both internally and externally in extract form.

SINUSITIS

Sinusitis is a condition involving inflammation and infection of the sinuses. It commonly affects the frontal and maxillary sinuses. The sinuses contain mucous membranes that moisten, filter, and warm the air as it enters the body and goes to the lungs. When they are clogged, drainage is inhibited and congestion results.

Sinusitis usually is a complication following less serious problems such as colds, hay fever and allergies. This may cause the area to become blocked and congested allowing for a bacterial infection. A sinus infection can be very uncomfortable, with symptoms such as a headache, earache, toothache, facial pain, sinus pressure, tenderness of the sinus areas, fever, and loss of smell. A child may be in severe pain, unable to distinguish the exact area where the pain is centered. The nasal area may be swollen.

CAUSES

A sinus infection occurs when the outlets for the sinuses become congested, irritated and inflamed. Mucus and air may build up causing pressure, pain and bacterial invasion. Bacterial sinusitis is usually caused by an upper respiratory infection from a cold or flu. Allergies and hayfever also make a child more susceptible to sinusitis. Some other factors which may contribute include environmental pollutants, dental infections, swimming and diving, cigarette smoke, or nasal abnormalities.

Some natural health professionals advocate keeping the colon in good functioning order. If the bowels are clogged, toxins can build up in the body, leading to disorders such as sinusitis. It is important to make sure the child gets plenty of fiber and fluid in the diet to ensure proper elimination.

HOME CARE

- A saline solution can be sprayed into the nasal passages.
- Encourage the child to rest to regain strength to fight the infection.
- Help the child blow his nose properly. Blow gently with both nostrils open for the best affect.
- A cool mist humidifier can help keep the sinuses draining properly.
- Fluids should be encouraged to help thin the mucus.
- Warm packs to the nasal area can reduce pain and encourage drainage.
- Soft ice packs and warm packs can be alternated to relieve discomfort and shrink inflammation.
- Avoid antihistimines if possible, because they may inhibit the mucus from being secreted.
- Treating colds naturally may help avoid secondary infections such as sinusitis.
- A hot ginger footbath can help draw the blood from the head to the feet to relieve congestion.

DIETARY GUIDELINES

- Fluid intake should be increased. Pure water, diluted fruit juices, and warm herbal teas are recommended.
- Warm soups such as chicken noodle and vegetable are recommended for helping congestion.
- Avoid all dairy products, especially if an allergy is suspected. They are mucus forming.
- Avoid refined sugar and food products as they may inhibit the healing process.
- Encourage a healthy diet of fruits, vegetables and whole grains.

NUTRITIONAL SUPPLEMENTS

- **Vitamin C and Bioflavonoids:** These are healing and will strengthen the immune system, reduce inflammation and fight infection.
- **Vitamin A/Beta-Carotene:** These are helpful in boosting the immune function and in healing the mucous membranes.
- **Zinc:** Lozenges and supplements can be used to heal for short periods of time, up to one week. Follow dosage directions.
- **B-Complex:** These will help with the infection.

HERBAL REMEDIES

- **Garlic:** Garlic has antibacterial properties to help fight the infection. Extracts can be given to children. Odorless capsules are also available.
- **Golden Seal:** Golden Seal has antibiotic properties which help fight infection.
- **Echinacea:** This can boost immune function and fight infection.

220

- **Comfrey and Fenugreek:** These help promote mucus flow in the upper respiratory system.
- **Eucalyptus:** This can help soothe inflammation and open nasal passages. It can be added to steam inhalations. A pack can be put over the sinus area.
- **Mullein:** This is soothing to inflamed tissue.
- **Aloe Vera:** Aloe helps in healing damaged tissue.

SORE THROAT / STREP THROAT

A sore throat refers to a painful sensation usually in the back of the throat, especially when swallowing. The throat, (pharynx), is a tube that separates into the breathing and digestive tracts. A sore throat is very common in children, occurring often during the winter and early spring. The degree of pain does not always determine the severity of the condition. Many different problems are associated with a sore throat. Pain that accompanies swollen lymph glands could be either viral or bacterial in nature. A sore throat may also occur with a head cold, runny nose, or ear infection. A simple sore throat will usually only last a few days.

CAUSES

Most sore throats are caused by either a virus or bacteria. Some other contributing factors may be cigarette smoke, environmental pollutants, allergies, fumes, hot foods, abrasions, dust, dry air, or screaming. Illnesses which often cause sore throats include tonsillitis, strep throat, pharyngitis, colds, influenza, laryngitis, mononucleosis, measles, mumps, and chicken pox. Strep throat is caused by the Streptococcal bacteria. Scarlet fever is characterized by a red rash. Left untreated, it may lead to rheumatic fever and heart valve damage. Strep throat is most often seen in children and up to one third of sore throats diagnosed are strep in nature. Some children carry the strep bacteria without actually having strep throat. It is best to treat the infection naturally if possible.

Home Care

- Fluid intake should be increased. Pure water, warm herbal teas, and soups are recommended.
- Use citrus juices such as orange, grapefruit, lime and lemon juice.
- Treat naturally at the first sign of illness to avoid secondary problems that may occur.
- Rest should be encouraged. A child needs to relax and lay down to allow the body to heal.
- If strep is suspected, consult a medical professional.
- A gargle can be made using 1/4 t. sea salt, four ounces of pure water, a t. of honey and a t. of squeezed lemon juice.
- Fruit juice popsicles may soothe the throat.
- A soft ice bag can be placed over a towel on the throat to relieve inflammation and reduce pain.
- A cool mist humidifier can help prevent sore throats.
- Using a stiff bristle brush, gently tap the gland area on the side of the throat. This can help increase blood circulation to the area and speed healing.
- Watch for signs of scarlet fever and rheumatic fever which may accompany strep throat.

Dietary Guidelines

- Fluid intake should be increased. Diluted citrus juices, carrot juice, herbal teas, and soups are recommended. Children can easily become dehydrated and the fluid will help dilute the mucus and eliminate toxins from the body.

- Avoid dairy products and refined carbohydrates and sugars.
- Fruit juice popsicles can help temporarily reduce pain and inflammation.
- Encourage a natural food diet with a lot of fruits, vegetables, and whole grains.

NUTRITIONAL SUPPLEMENTS

- **Vitamin C and Bioflavonoids:** These will help heal the tissue, improve immune function, reduce inflammation, and heal the infection.
- **Vitamin A/Beta-Carotene:** Vitamin A and Beta-Carotene can help boost immune function and aid in healing the mucous membranes.
- **Zinc:** Lozenges can help soothe and promote tissue healing. They should not be taken longer than a week, and follow the recommended dosage.
- **Chlorophyll:** A Chlorophyll drink can help encourage healing and cleaning of toxins from the body.
- **Acidophilus and Bifidus:** Acidophilus is important, especially if antibiotics are being taken, to return beneficial bacteria to the digestive tract.
- **Indoles:** Dietary indoles can help strengthen the immune system.

HERBAL REMEDIES

- **Echinacea:** This is a natural antibiotic helpful in fighting both viral and bacterial infections and in boosting the immune system.
- **Golden Seal:** Another great herb to help fight infection.
- **Garlic:** Garlic can help fight infection because of its natural antibiotic properties. Odorless capsules or extracts can be used for children.

223

- **Yarrow:** This can promote sweating and aid in reducing fever.
- **Chamomile:** Chamomile tea may help soothe the throat and relax the child.
- **Hyssop:** Hyssop works to heal the throat and fight infection.
- **Catnip:** This will help heal and relax.
- **Hops:** A nervine herb to help relax the child and speed healing.
- **Lobelia:** Lobelia can help relax the body and relieve congestion.

STOMACHACHE

A stomachache can occur in a child at any age for a myriad of reasons. They are common during the childhood years and are rarely serious.

CAUSES

A stomachache can be caused by a number of conditions such as nervousness, worrying, food poisoning, eating too much, constipation, eating too fast, medication, food allergies, additives, or even environmental pollutants. Watch the child to see if other symptoms are present. If it lasts more than a few hours and there is a fever, nausea, diarrhea, vomiting, or headache, it may be a more serious condition and a medical professional should be consulted.

Food allergies are a common cause of stomachaches in children. Cow's milk is often not tolerated by children and can make them uncomfortable and suffer pain.

HOME CARE

- Make the child as comfortable as possible.
- A hot water bottle on the stomach may help ease the discomfort.
- Try to see if the child is suffering from emotional concerns that may be causing the stomachache.
- If the conditions worsens or other symptoms appear, check with a medical professional.
- If vomiting or diarrhea are present, protect against possible dehydration.

DIETARY GUIDELINES

- Offer sips of pure water or ice chips.
- Clear liquids should only be given if the child is vomiting.

NUTRITIONAL SUPPLEMENTS

- **Acidophilus and Bifidus:** Acidophilus will help with digestion and in restoring beneficial bacterial into the digestive tract.

HERBAL REMEDIES

- **Chamomile:** Chamomile tea can help relax the child and ease stomach discomfort.
- **Peppermint:** Peppermint tea is soothing for the stomach and digestion.
- **Ginger:** Ginger tea or capsules are very effective for nausea, vomiting and stomach complaints.

- **Aloe Vera:** The gel can help ease and resolve stomach problems.
- **Catnip:** This is mild and soothing as a tea for children.

STRESS

It is sad but true that many children suffer from stress related complaints. Family problems, abuse, tension, violence, fear, school pressures, and many other concerns cause stress in children. There are small children suffering from depression in our society. They feel the adult stress and pressures as they are rushed from place to place. Stress related emotional and medical problems have increased in the past few decades.

CAUSES

Stress can be the result of various factors in children. Divorce, death of a loved one, school pressures, fear of violence, physical threats, along with many more, may cause stress in a child. Symptoms include headaches, ulcers, diarrhea, loss of appetite, fatigue, asthma, rashes, and lowered immune response.

When the body remains in a stressful situation for prolonged periods of time, it can react by increasing adrenaline which elevates the heart rate, shuts down digestion, and increases respiration. Internalizing stress can cause a child to suffer mental and physical problems.

A lack of essential nutrients can cause a weakened immune system. A low immune response causes the nervous system to not function properly during times of stress. A strong nervous system is essential in handling stressful situations that occur.

Helping a child deal with stress is vital. Negative emotions have a harmful effect on children. Try to make the home a place of refuge and peace. Children need down time when they can just lay around and relax without feeling pressured to do something. Laughter has a positive effect on body functions. Make home time enjoyable and being together fun. Create a balance in the life of a child between school, friends, family relations, religious beliefs, recreation, and self-worth.

HOME CARE

- Encourage exercise regularly. Physical activity releases endorphins in the brain that promote a sense of well being and can reduce tension.
- Practice deep breathing with the child. Exhale completely through the mouth slowly. Inhale through the nose counting to four. Exhale slowly and completely. Repeat three times.
- Play soothing, classical music around the house when the child is feeling stressed.
- Avoid television programs that may frighten the child.
- Listen to the child's concerns and fears. Let them talk about their problems without feeling criticism.
- Make sure the child is getting enough sleep. They require more sleep than adults and should be encouraged to have a regular bedtime.
- Seek professional help if the problem continues.

DIETARY GUIDELINES

- Avoid giving a child chocolate, caffeine, soda, refined sugars and products, fatty foods, junk food and fried foods. These can heighten the stress response.

- Encourage a diet with nutritional value. Fruits, vegetables and whole grains should be emphasized.
- Make sure children eat regular meals. They need the food to help blood sugar levels.
- A nutritious diet helps to keep the adrenal glands functioning properly, and they are directly responsible for stress reactions.

NUTRITIONAL SUPPLEMENTS

- **B-Complex Vitamins:** The B-Complex vitamins are essential for maintaining good mental health. They are known as the stress vitamins and work on the nervous system. Many children are lacking in B-vitamins which are used up more quickly when the body is under stress.
- **Vitamin E:** Vitamin E helps protect the glands during stress.
- **Vitamin C and Bioflavonoids:** These can help stimulate adrenal function which may be suppressed during prolonged stress.
- **Calcium and Magnesium:** This combination helps calm the nervous system.

HERBAL REMEDIES

- **Chamomile:** Chamomile tea can help relax a child before bedtime.
- **Passion Flower:** This is a natural tranquilizer to relax the body and mind. It may not be suitable for young children.
- **Lobelia:** Lobelia can be used in extract form to help relaxation.

SUDDEN INFANT DEATH SYNDROME

Sudden infant death syndrome (SIDS) is the leading cause of infant death between the ages of one month and one year in the United States. The peak age for SIDS is two to four months. Winter is the most common time for deaths to occur. There are no visible signs to predict this syndrome. The babies seem normal and healthy. The tragedy is extremely painful for the families involved.

CAUSES

The cause of SIDS is not known but there are some theories. It appears that some factors may increase the chances of a baby dying from SIDS. Some include low birth weight, premature birth, siblings of SIDS babies, mothers who abused drugs during pregnancy, babies from poor families, young mothers, high lead levels in blood, vaccinations, cigarette smoking in the home, and laying a baby on their stomach. Though in many cases none of these factors are involved, it is important to protect the infant from possible problems.

The sleeping position of infants has been studied. It used to be that pediatricians recommended that infants sleep on their stomachs to avoid gagging or choking, in case they vomit while sleeping. But studies done by various individuals, including one conducted by Dr. Warren Guntheroth of the University of Washington Medical Center, found that infants put on their backs to sleep had a lower risk of SIDS death. Since infants often suffer from mild pauses in breathing, known as apneas, lying on the back allows them to recover easier through catching their breath and gasping.

Breast fed babies are at less of a risk for SIDS. Harris L. Coulter and Barbara Loe Fisher in their book *A Shot In The*

Dark suggest that the pertussis vaccine given to infants at ages two, four and six months may contribute to the SIDS deaths.

HOME CARE

- Breast feed if possible. This is recommended by health and medical professionals for the best method of feeding an infant.
- Put the child to sleep laying on their backs. This is new advice during the past few years.

DIETARY GUIDELINES

- Mothers should eat a healthy diet during pregnancy such as natural foods, including fruits, vegetables and whole grains.
- Avoid chemical additives during pregnancy.

NUTRITIONAL SUPPLEMENTS

- **Vitamin A:** This is needed especially after the first three months.
- **Vitamin C and Bioflavonoids:** If the mother is nursing, she can take a supplement. Babies can take a liquid supplement, according to directions on the label.

HERBAL REMEDIES

- **Red Raspberry:** This is recommended during pregnancy.

SUNBURN

A sunburn can take the fun out of any vacation. It's easy to forget sun protection when having a great time. A sunburn involves the outer layers of the skin and it is usually a first degree burn. A second degree burn occurs if blisters and swelling develop which means the dermis has been affected. A child's skin is tender and can easily burn. It should be protected from the sun's rays. Infants and babies need even more protection because sun screens are not recommended for them. Keep babies out of the sun or under an umbrella. It should be noted that they can even burn in the shade, but it is less likely. So watch them carefully.

CAUSES

Sunburns occur from exposure to radiation from the sun. It comes in the form of ultraviolet rays, UVB and UVA, which are both harmful.

HOME CARE

- Apply sunscreen when children will be in the sun for any extended length of time.
- A hat and sunglasses are also recommended.
- Gradually expose children to the sun.
- Children can burn even on cloudy days.
- Fair skinned children are more susceptible to burning.
- A cool bath can ease the discomfort.

DIETARY GUIDELINES

- Fluids should be encouraged, as dehydration can occur with excessive exposure to the sun.

NUTRITIONAL GUIDELINES

- **Vitamin A/Beta-Carotene:** These can help heal the skin.
- **Vitamin C and Bioflavonoids:** These are important in immune function and the healing process.

HERBAL REMEDIES

- **Aloe Vera:** Aloe vera gel can be applied directly to the affected area. It can help heal and soothe the skin after a burn and has been used as a treatment for centuries.

TEETHING

Teething has been blamed for many different complaints in infants. If they have a runny nose, are cranky, or awaken during the night, many believe it is due to teething. Teething is not an illness and as with most minor ailments in infants, the symptoms usually disappear naturally and quickly. Babies begin the teething process at many different ages. The bottom center teeth are most often the first to appear around six months. But it is not unusual for others to appear first. Teething is a very individual development. The first sign is a small bump on the gum from which a tooth should emerge within two weeks. The back molars should appear at about one to three years of age. The complete set of twenty baby teeth are usually all in by three years of age.

Permanent teeth usually begin to push through around six years of age. Fortunately, they don't cause the same irritation as the baby teeth and usually proceed with little problem.

Some of the symptoms associated with teething include ear rubbing, crying for no reason, slight fever, drooling, chewing on hard objects, runny nose, waking at night, and restlessness. A baby who is teething will chew on anything including the crib, toys, and fingers.

CAUSES

Teething follows the normal pattern of tooth development. The pain and irritation is the result of the pressure from the crown of the tooth against the gums. Once the tooth breaks through the gum membrane, the pain and irritation usually subside.

HOME CARE

- The gums can be massaged with a fingertip to relieve discomfort.
- Allow the infant to chew on something hard.
- Keep some teething rings in the refrigerator. Cold objects help numb the gum surface to relieve discomfort temporarily.
- A cool, damp, clean cloth can be used to chew on.

DIETARY GUIDELINES

- Raw carrots, celery, and raw apples can be chewed on, but make sure the child is in a sitting position and that they don't gnaw off a piece and choke.
- Avoid rich foods as they interfere with digestion.
- Breast feeding can continue, and the baby may want to nurse more often.

NUTRITIONAL SUPPLEMENTS

- **Calcium:** A liquid calcium supplement can be given. Some believe this can help the teething process.
- **Multi-Mineral Supplement:** Minerals may be lacking.
- **Vitamin D:** This will help with the absorption of important minerals.

HERBAL REMEDIES

- **Chamomile:** Chamomile tea will help relax the baby and ease the pain.
- **Catnip:** Catnip tea can help calm the infant.
- **Lobelia:** Lobelia can be rubbed on the gums and back to promote relaxation and relieve pain.

THRUSH

Thrush is a fungal infection of the mouth. It is a very common ailment with no dangerous side effects. It is caused by the fungus Candida albicans which also causes some forms of diaper rash and vaginal yeast infections. Stet is most commonly seen in infants under six months of age.

Thrush is characterized by thick, white, cloudy spots in the mouth, sides of the cheeks and tongue. It may cause some discomfort for the baby and he may be irritable. It may also affect the diaper area with a rash with red pimple-like spots and inflammation.

It can take a while for the condition to clear up. If the thrush occurs with a fever, cough or other symptoms, consult a physician.

CAUSES

Thrush is caused by the fungus Candida albicans. It should be treated to avoid a chronic problem.

HOME CARE

- Nursing mothers should make sure their diet is free of refined sugar and white flour products. Yeast thrives on these.
- Do not attempt to pick off patches of the white thrush. This can cause bleeding and may lead to a secondary infection.

DIETARY GUIDELINES

- Breast feeding mothers should avoid refined sugar products, white flour products, and fatty foods. These inhibit the healing process and allow for yeast to thrive.
- If breast feeding, eat a natural, nutritious diet.

NUTRITIONAL SUPPLEMENTS

- **Acidophilus and Bifidus:** This should be taken by nursing mothers to encourage the growth of the beneficial bacteria and inhibit the growth of the fungus. It can also be given to the infant in liquid form diluted with water; 1/4 t. to 1/2 cup water. Use an eyedropper.
- **Indoles:** Dietary indoles help strengthen the immune system.
- If nursing, include supplements of the antioxidant vitamins such as **vitamin C, E, Beta-carotene, zinc, and selenium.**

HERBAL REMEDIES

- **Aloe Vera:** Aloe Vera gel has antifungal properties. Dip your finger in the gel and apply to the affected area.
- **Garlic:** Odorless Garlic can be taken by the nursing mother.
- **Ginger:** Ginger contains antibacterial and antifungal properties. A nursing mother can drink ginger tea or take a capsule.

TOOTH DECAY

Tooth decay is a condition in which the enamel and dentin of the teeth gradually disintegrate. It takes months or even years for the bacterial plaque to dissolve the tooth. If the decay continues, it can enter the tubules toward the pulp causing infection. In order for decay to occur, the bacteria must be present for a period of time and the child must be susceptible to decay. It appears that certain children are more prone to this condition. Tooth decay will not be apparent until it is in an advanced state, and it may be sensitive to heat or cold.

Though some children are more susceptible, conditions can either promote or reduce the possibility of tooth decay.

CAUSES

Tooth decay is caused by the build up of plaque on the surface of the teeth which, over a prolonged period of time, causes the enamel and dentin of the teeth to dissolve. For tooth decay to occur, bacteria must be present which cause the problem and the child must be susceptible to tooth decay. For this to occur certain conditions must be present such as poor tooth enamel, imbalances in the blood, poor mineral assimilation, acidic saliva, or a poor diet. Foods which can aid in tooth decay include refined sugars, dairy products, acidic foods, soda, refined starches, and excessive fruit juice consumption. Children who drink a lot of soda can have excessive amounts of phosphorus which can lead to calcium deficiency.

HOME CARE

- A dentist should be consulted if decay is suspected. Choose a dentist who is used to working with children and is kind, soft spoken and gentle.
- Encourage children to brush their teeth carefully.
- Avoid giving a baby fruit juice in a bottle. Hold off until he can drink from a cup.
- Do not give the child sweets before bedtime. This includes fruit and fruit juices.

DIETARY GUIDELINES

- Avoid refined sugars, soda, excessive amounts of fruit juice, fats and refined carbohydrates.
- Encourage a healthy diet with natural, whole foods such as fruits, vegetables and whole grains.
- Avoid sticky, sugary foods that stick to the teeth.
- Goat's milk, avocados, garlic, oats, brown rice, cabbage, greens, parsley and endive provide natural fluoride to strengthen the teeth.
- Eating healthy foods during pregnancy helps to ensure proper development of teeth.

NUTRITIONAL SUPPLEMENTS

- **Vitamin C:** Avoid chewable vitamin C which can destroy the enamel on the teeth. Have the child suck the tablet or give liquid vitamin C.
- **Calcium and Magnesium:** These help with teeth development.
- **Multi-Mineral Supplement:** Minerals help with all body functions including structural development.

HERBAL REMEDIES

- **Chamomile:** Chamomile tea can be given before a visit to the dentist to help the child relax.
- **Oatstraw:** This contains silica which helps in the development of strong bones and teeth.
- **Calcium herbal formulas** are beneficial which contain horsetail and oatstraw.

TOXIC METAL SYNDROME

Children are at risk for exposure to toxins from the home and environment. Approximately fifty cancer-causing substances, including lead, mercury and nickel have been found in ground water in twenty-six states. Toxic metals are systemic poisons which inhibit biochemical enzyme function and can cause malfunctions in the body. Children breathe the same air that adults breathe with the same level of pollutants. And children actually breathe in more air than adults in relation to their body weight. Children also eat more than adults in relation to their body weight and are exposed to more toxins found in foods, such as residue of pesticides and additives. A child's immune system is not as efficient as an adult's which helps to rid the body of the toxins.

Lead is a major contributor to Toxic Metal Syndrome. Since this problem has been recognized by many, the incidents have lessened. But there are still as many as fifteen percent of children tested in some areas that have toxic levels of lead. Lead tends to accumulate in the immune system, brain and kidneys and can cause severe functional disorders. Some of the problems associated with lead poisoning include mental retardation, learning disabilities, low IQ, vision problems, high blood pressure, stroke, kidney disease, coordination difficulties and hyperactivity. Lead is in the air we breathe and children living in a large city environment are at higher risk. Pregnant women who work with lead in industrial jobs have been found to have higher incidence of birth defects, infertility, miscarriage and premature births.

Mercury is also a problem. It is actually more toxic than lead and is found in the soil, water, seafood, fungicides and pesticides. Mercury is also found in dental fillings and minute amounts have been found to leak from the fillings and enter the brain. For this reason, many health-conscious individuals choose a dentist who can fill cavities with material other than silver fillings which contain mercury. Mercury can cause insomnia, dizziness, fatigue, dermatitis, brain function disorders and depression.

Nickel is another toxic metal. It is found in water, processed foods, fertilizers and tobacco smoke. Conditions associated with nickel poisoning include nervous system disorders, epilepsy, stroke, toxemia and cancer.

Arsenic is a highly toxic metal often found in water, pesticides, seafood, tobacco smoke, laundry detergents, pollution from industry and exhaust and even beer. Those at high risk are individuals who work with pesticides and insecticides, miners, metal workers, and copper smelters. The poisoning primarily centers on the lungs, skin and liver. It can cause headaches, brain disorders, confusion, vomiting, diarrhea, and convulsions. A hair analysis can help to determine if toxic levels are in the system.

Cadmium is another toxic trace mineral. It can replace the body's reserves of zinc in the kidneys and liver. High levels in the body can cause high blood pressure, anemia, joint disorders, hair loss, kidney and liver disorders, cancer and loss of appetite. It can weaken the immune system and lead to many disorders. Cigarette smokers often have elevated levels of cadmium.

CAUSES

Toxic Metal Syndrome can be caused by exposure to lead, mercury, nickel, aluminum, arsenic, cadmium and other toxic metals through breathing, pollution, car emissions, dental fillings, food, pesticides, additives, and drinking water.

HOME CARE

- Have drinking water tested for toxic metals.
- Eat organically grown foods.
- A hair analysis can identify metal toxicity.

DIETARY GUIDELINES

- Drink plenty of distilled or pure water.
- Eat organically grown foods.
- Onions, garlic and beans add sulfur to help rid the body of toxins.
- Eat a high fiber diet to help keep the colon functioning well.
- Eat foods high in sulfur such as eggs, onions, garlic, beans and legumes. Sulfur helps the body to eliminate arsenic.

Nutritional Supplements

- **Vitamin A:** This is helpful in eliminating toxic metals found in chemicals in food, air and water.
- **B-Complex:** B-Complex vitamins help protect the immune system to prevent cellular damage.
- **Vitamin C and Bioflavonoids:** These work together to protect the immune system. They help increase the strength of the capillary walls and protect them against toxic poisoning.
- **Calcium:** Calcium helps to prevent accumulation of lead in the bones.
- **Germanium:** Germanium has been found to actually bind with toxic metals and prevent them from being dispersed in the body.
- **Zinc:** Zinc helps to eliminate toxic metals and strengthen the immune system.
- **CoQ10:** This helps protect the immune system and aids in oxygenating the cells to resist stress and disease.
- **Chlorophyll/Blue-Green Algae:** This is a natural cleanser for the blood stream.
- **Indoles:** Dietary indoles help strengthen the immune system.

Herbal Remedies

- **Garlic:** Garlic is a natural antibiotic and contains germanium and selenium which work to neutralize toxic metals.
- **Ginkgo:** This is a strong antioxidant to help the immune system. It improves memory and mental function.
- **Gotu Kola:** This is food for the brain and helps to build energy reserves and protect the body against toxic buildup.
- **Kelp:** Kelp helps to bind with metals such as lead and

flush them from the body.
*   **Sulfur Herbs:** These help to protect the body from heavy metal toxicity. Some include Horseradish, Watercress, Alfalfa, Burdock, Dandelion, Comfrey, Garlic, Onions, Sarsaparilla, Kelp, Echinacea, Lobelia, Mullein, Parsley, Cayenne, Chaparral, and Nettle.

URINARY TRACT INFECTION

Urinary tract infections are caused by a bacteria in the urethra, ureters, kidneys or bladder. Bladder infections are the most common. Young children or infants with a urinary tract infection may not be able to express what they are feeling. Most often there is a burning sensation especially when urinating, painful and frequent urination, dark urine, foul odor in urine, fever, backache, loss of appetite, and there may be blood in the urine. Females are more susceptible to urinary tract infections because of their anatomy. The urethra lies close to the rectum where bacteria can get into the urinary tract. The condition is more serious if it involves the kidneys, but this is rare.

CAUSES

Urinary tract infections are most often caused by bacteria normally present in bowel movements. The bacteria is normally washed out through the urine if the bladder is functioning well. Food allergies have been known to cause recurring problems with urinary tract infections. The sensitivity can cause the bladder to become irritated and more susceptible to infection. Bubble baths have also been associated with this condition. Girls especially are more vulnerable because of the short distance between the urethra and bladder. Other factors include: dyes in clothing, scented and dyed toilet paper, detergents, soaps, poor hygiene, yeast infections, pinworms and injury.

HOME CARE

- Use white, untreated toilet paper.
- Girls, especially, should wear cotton, white underwear to avoid problems.
- Encourage good hygiene.
- Girls should be taught to wipe from front to back to avoid infection.

DIETARY GUIDELINES

- Many studies have shown that cranberry juice contains properties which hinder the bacteria from adhering to the bladder wall. Choose cranberry juice without added refined sugar for the best results. Dilute for younger children.
- Fluid intake should be increased. Pure water can help flush the bacteria from the urinary system.
- Limit refined sugars, processed foods, and fatty foods as they can interfere with the healing process.
- Encourage a nutritious diet with fruits, vegetables, and whole grains.

NUTRITIONAL SUPPLEMENTS

- **Acidophilus and Bifidus:** Acidophilus can help by increasing the presence of beneficial bacteria. This is especially helpful when antibiotic therapy is used.

- **Vitamin C and Bioflavonoids:** Vitamin C can help reduce inflammation and speed the healing process.
- **Vitamin A/Beta-Carotene:** These can help boost the immune function, soothe mucous membranes, and aid in healing.

HERBAL REMEDIES

- **Cranberries:** Numerous studies have shown the healing effects of cranberries on the urinary tract. Cranberry juice or cranberry capsules can be used.
- **Garlic:** Garlic is a natural antibiotic to kill the bacteria associated with the infection. Odorless capsules or an extract can be used.
- **Uva Ursi:** This has been used for centuries in treating urinary tract infections. It has antiseptic and astringent properties. It should not be given to children under six and is usually found in combination with other herbs.
- **Echinacea:** This helps boost the immune system and speed the healing process.
- **Golden Seal:** Golden Seal is beneficial for its antibacterial properties and is soothing to the mucous membranes.
- **Use an herbal formula** for the urinary tract and kidneys.

VACCINATIONS
(See chapter on immunizations)

WARTS

Warts are unpleasant, no matter what the age of the child. They are usually circular, raised, rough skin growths commonly seen on children. They are harmless and caused by a virus. Warts are most often seen on the hands, arms and legs but may also appear on the neck, face and genital area.

They can occur at any age but usually between the ages of ten and seventeen. Girls seem to be more often affected than boys. Warts seem to be able to spread from one part of the body to another but are rarely spread from person to person. They usually do not cause pain unless they are scratched or injured. Warts generally disappear within a few years on their own. They can be removed by a physician if a child is particularly sensitive.

The most common type of wart is Verruca vulgaris. It is the typical round, raised with rough surface type. Plantar warts occur on the bottom of the feet but are less prevalent.

CAUSES

Warts are caused by viruses resulting in the harmless growths.

HOME CARE

• If the child is not bothered, ignore the problem. They will usually spontaneously disappear within a few years.
• Children are sometimes tempted to pick at the wart. This can cause infection and perhaps spreading and should be avoided.

DIETARY GUIDELINES

- Limit refined sugars, processed foods and fatty foods. This can encourage viral growth.
- A healthy diet is important for all children. Encourage fruits, vegetables and whole grains. Green and yellow vegetables contain vitamins and minerals healing to the skin.

NUTRITIONAL SUPPLEMENTS

- **Vitamin A:** This can be taken internally or squeezed out and applied to the wart.
- **Beta-Carotene:** This boosts immune function and helps with healing.
- **Vitamin E:** Vitamin E can be taken internally and applied directly to the wart. It is an antioxidant and helps the immune system.
- **Vitamin C:** Vitamin C helps boost the immune function.

HERBAL REMEDIES

- **Tea Tree Oil:** Tea Tree oil can be applied directly to the wart.
- **Dandelion:** The stem of the Dandelion can be opened and rubbed on the wart to heal.
- **Honey:** Honey has antiviral properties and is an old remedy for healing warts.
- **Banana:** The peel of a banana can be rubbed on a wart. It may be taped in place as well.

WHOOPING COUGH

The medical term for whooping cough is Bordetella pertussis. A vaccine is commonly administered to babies beginning at the age of two months. Though controversial, there has been a decrease in the number of whooping cough cases in the United States. But in recent years, a resurgence to some degree has occurred.

Whooping cough usually begins as an apparent common respiratory infection or cold. The cough usually worsens with a deep inhalation and whooping sound. Vomiting, excess mucus, exhaustion and anxiety may also appear. The cough may continue for up to six weeks.

This condition can be very serious for infants and small children. They may suffer from oxygen deprivation, dehydration, convulsions or hemorrhage. Ear infections and pneumonia may appear as secondary infections. Children suspected of having whooping cough should be given medical attention.

CAUSES

Whooping cough is caused by the bacteria Bordetella pertussis. It is spread from person to person via the respiratory tract from coughing, sneezing, breathing, or sharing eating utensils. The incubation period is usually just under ten days but may appear anywhere from five to twenty-one days after exposure.

HOME CARE

- Isolate a child with whooping cough to avoid exposure to other family members and friends. This should continue for up to one month after the onset of the disease.

- A medical professional should be consulted if whooping cough is suspected, as it is a serious condition, especially for infants and small children.
- If a child is having difficulty breathing, seek medical attention.
- Rest is essential, and exercise may induce coughing attacks.
- If the weather is nice, a child may benefit from a few minutes of resting in the sun.

DIETARY GUIDELINES

- Fluid intake is important to avoid dehydration and to help dilute mucus secretions. Pure water, herbal teas, diluted fruit juices, home-made vegetable and grain soups, and fruit juice popsicles can be given.
- Avoid dairy products and fatty foods as they may increase mucus production.
- Encourage a diet full of nutritious foods such as fruits, vegetables and whole grains.

NATURAL SUPPLEMENTS

- **Vitamin C and Bioflavonoids:** These work to increase immune function, reducing inflammation, and aid in healing.
- **Vitamin A/Beta-Carotene:** These are important to help the immune system and heal mucous membranes.
- **Acidophilus and Bifidus:** These help with bowel function and promote the growth of beneficial bacteria.
- **Zinc:** Zinc helps boost immune function and aids in healing. Follow recommended dosage.
- **Indoles:** Dietary indoles work to strengthen the immune system.

Herbal Remedies

- **Slippery Elm:** Slippery elm bark is soothing to the mucous membranes.
- **Marshmallow:** Marshmallow is soothing and healing to the respiratory tract.
- **Garlic:** This contains antibacterial properties for healing. It can be given in extract or odorless capsules.
- **Echinacea:** This helps immune function and in the healing process.
- **Chamomile:** Chamomile tea promotes relaxation.
- **Licorice:** Licorice tea or extract has antibacterial properties and is soothing to the respiratory tract.

GENERAL BIBLIOGRAPHY FOR FURTHER READING

Aihara, Cornellia, *Macrobiotic Child Care*. Oroville, CA: George Ohsawa Macrobiotic Foundation, 1979.

Austin, Phylis, *Natural Healthcare For Your Child*. Sunfield, MI: Family Health Publications, 1990.

Balch, James F. M.D. and Phyllis A. Balch, C.N.C., *Prescription For Nutritional Healing*. Garden City Park, N.Y: Avery Publishing, 1990.

Challem, Jack Joseph, *Let's Live*, Sept. 1990.

Cooper, Robert Ph.D., *Health and Fitness Excellence*. Boston: Houghton Mifflin Company, 1989.

Coulter, Harris L. and Barbara Loe Fisher, *A Shot In The Dark*. Garden City Park, N.Y.: Avery Publishing Group, Inc.

Davidson, Joan, "Singing Low-Down Sugar Blues." *Chimo*, 12/81.

Elkins, Rita, *The Complete Home Health Advisor*. Pleasant Grove, UT: Woodland Publishing Co., 1994.

Galland, Leo. M.D., *Superimmunity for Kids*. New York: Delta, 1988.

Gamble, John, *Vaccination -exploring some myths*.

Gooch, Sandy, *If You Love Me Don't Feed Me Junk*! Reston, Virginia: Reston Publishing Company, Inc. 1983.

Hill, Barbara Albers, *Baby Tactics*. Garden City Par, N.Y: Avery Publishing Group Inc., 1991.

Hoekelman, Robert, M.D., Noni Macdonald, M.D. and David Baum, M.D., *The New American Encyclopedia of Children's Health*. New York: New American Library, 1989.

Horne, Steven H., *The ABC Herbal*. Winona Lake, Indiana: Wendall Whitman Company, 1992.

Lieberman, Shari, and Nancy Bruning. *The Real Vitamin and Mineral Book*. Garden City, NY: Avery Publishing Group, 1990.

Marti, James E., *Alternative Health Medicine Encyclopedia.* Detroit: Visible Ink Press, 1995.

Mendelsohn, Robert S. M.D., *How To Have A Healthy Child In Spite of Your Doctor.* Chicago: Contemporary Books, 1984.

Murray, Michael T. N.D., *The Healing Power of Herbs.* Rocklin, CA: Prima Publishing, 1995.

Murray, Michael T. N.D. and Joseph Pizzorno, N.D., *Encyclopedia of Natural Medicine.* Rocklin, CA: Prima Publishing, 1991.

Ody, Penelope, *The Complete Medicinal Herbal.* New York: Dorling Kindersley, Inc., 1993.

Pantell, Robert H. M.D., James F. Fries, M.D. and Donald M. Vickery, M.D., *Taking Care of Your Child.* Reading, Massachusetts: Addison-Wesley Publishing Company, 1977.

Ritchason, Jack, *The Little Herb Encyclopedia.* Pleasant Grove, UT: Woodland Publishing Inc., 1994.

Ritchason, Jack, *Vitamin and Health Encyclopedia.* Pleasant Grove, UT: Woodland Publishing Inc., 1994.

Schauss, Alexander, *Prevention,* October, 1983.

Schwab, Dr. Laurence, *Let's Live,* Jan. 1984.

Simone, Charles, *Cancer and Nutrition.* Garden City Park, NY: Avery Publishing Group, 1992.

Smith, Lendon, *Feed Your Kids Right.* New York: Dell Publishing, 1979.

Smith, Lendon, *Improving Your Child's Behavior Chemistry.* Englewood Cliffs, New Jersy: Prentice-Hall, Inc., 1976.

Tenney, Deanne, *Introduction To Natural Health.* Pleasant Grove, UT: Woodland Publishing Inc., 1995.

Tenney, Deanne, *Natural Health Guide.* Pleasant Grove, UT: Woodland Publishing Inc., 1995.

Tenney, Louise, *The Encyclopedia of Natural Remedies.* Pleasant Grove, UT: Woodland Publishing Inc., 1995.

Tenney, Louise, *Health Handbook.* Pleasant Grove, UT: Woodland Publishing Inc., 1987.

Tenney, Louise, *Nutritional Guide With Food Combining*. Pleasant Grove, UT: Woodland Publishing Inc., 1991.

Tenney, Louise, *Today's Herbal Health*. Pleasant Grove, UT: Woodland Publishing Inc., 1992.

Toms, Laraine, *Cooking For Your Baby The Natural Way*. New York: Sterling Publishing Co., 1984.

Weber, Marcea, *Encyclopedia of Natural Health and Healing for Children*. Rocklin, CA: Prima Publishing, 1992.

Weil, Andrew, M.D., *Natural Health, Natural Medicine*. Boston: Houghton Mifflin Company, 1990.

Weiner, Michael A. Ph.D., *Healing Children Naturally*. San Rafael, CA: Quantum Books, 1993.

Weissbluth, Marc, M.D., *Healthy Sleep Habits, Happy Child*. New York: Fawcett Columbine, 1987.

Zand, Janet, LAc, O.M.D., Rachel Walton, R.N. and Bob Rountree, M.D., *Smart Medicine For A Healthier Child*. Garden City Park, N.Y: Avery Publishing, 1994.

INDEX